LABOR PAIN

A Natural Approach to Easing Delivery

Nicky Wesson

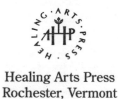

Healing Arts Press
Rochester, Vermont

Healing Arts Press
One Park Street
Rochester, Vermont 05767
www.InnerTraditions.com

Healing Arts Press is a division of Inner Traditions International

Copyright © 1999, 2000 by Nicky Wesson
Illustrations copyright (pages 63 and 64) © Random House UK Ltd 1999
Originally published in London by Vermilion

First U.S. edition published by Healing Arts Press in 2000

*Note to the reader: This book is intended as an informational guide. The
remedies, approaches, and techniques described herein are meant to
supplement, and not to be a substitute for, professional medical care or
treatment. They should not be used to treat a serious ailment without prior
consultation with a qualified health care professional.*

Library of Congress Cataloging-in-Publication Data

Wesson, Nicky.
    Labor pain : a natural approach to easing delivery / Nicky Wesson.—
1st U.S. ed.
        p. cm.
    Originally published: London : Vermilion, 1999.
    Includes bibliographical references and index.
    ISBN 0-89281-895-6 (alk. paper)
    1. Natural childbirth. 2. Therapeutics, Physiological. I. Title.

    RG661 .W456 2000
    618.4'5—dc21

                                                    99-461974

Printed and bound in Canada

10 9 8 7 6 5 4 3 2 1

This book was typeset in Century Old Style

CONTENTS

Acknowledgments iv

Introduction v

Chapter 1 The Process of Labor 1

Chapter 2 Pain 18

Chapter 3 Physiology of Labor 28

Chapter 4 Psychology of Labor 39

Chapter 5 Environment 46

Chapter 6 Preparing for Labor 54

Chapter 7 Positions in Labor 78

Chapter 8 Natural Aids to Pain Relief 86

Chapter 9 Drugs and Pain Relief 118

Chapter 10 Episiotomies and Tears 127

Chapter 11 Cesarean Section 131

Chapter 12 Postpartum Pain 136

References 141

Suggested Reading 147

Resources 149

Index 150

ACKNOWLEDGMENTS

I would like to thank all the people who have helped me with this book, including the many pregnant women whom I have spoken to over the years. I am particularly grateful to those who invited me to be present when they gave birth, which was a real honor and privilege – especially Nic and David.

Many people have been very generous with their time and information, in particular:

Sarah Leigh – for especial support and encouragement; Beverley Lawrence Beech; Linda Carpenter; Caroline Casterton; Pat Corben; Marie Coveney; Ros d'Albert; Joyce Dixon; Hazel Donavan; Nadine Edwards; Sue Francia; Christine Grabowska; the staff of Hampton Library; Karen Howell of the Old Operating Theatre and Herb Garret; Lorraine Jones of the Royal Pharmaceutical Society; Roy Kelly, Elaine McClelland and the staff of Richmond Library; Anna Knight; Paul Lewis; Anne Lunt; Beatsa Marshall; Tonie Neville; Margot Richardson; Elizabeth Rodgers; the Royal College of Midwives Library staff; Jane Shore; Alex Smith; Brenda Tebby; Sue Turner; Sharon van Klink; Roy Vickery and the Botanic Library staff; the Wellcome Institute Library staff.

Introduction

Many people have wondered why labor should be so painful, particularly when animals do not seem to find it so. There is no really obvious answer. Formerly, it was believed to be a punishment to be borne by all mothers to atone for Eve's sin in the Garden of Eden. Some people believe that labor pain signals the need to reach a safe place to have the baby, while others believe that it makes childbirth such a memorable event that you value your child more. The investment of labor carries you through caring for it for many years to come. Some feel that without pain there is no gain.

To some extent, it must be part of the price for being upright and walking on two feet instead of on all fours. The muscle power required to hold in 20 pounds of added weight of baby, placenta, fluid, and weighty uterus cannot be undone lightly. Indeed, when you consider the size of the baby and the relatively small area through which it has to pass, it is not surprising that it is painful. Yet some people find it more painful than others – for reasons that will be examined.

Labor *is* very painful. It can be hard to realize how much it can hurt even when it is entirely normal and is a natural physiological process that is going on all the time. In the West it has never been safer in terms of survival of mother and baby, previously a justifiable cause of anxiety for every pregnant woman. However, the medicalization that, in part, is responsible for the improved outlook for women may now also be making labor more painful, as normal birth without any obstetric intervention becomes increasingly rare.

Research is showing increasingly that the things that make the most difference to improving the outcome of labor are not technological advances, but feeling comfortable about the place in which you give birth and the human support that you have at the time.

Personal experience taught me the hard way that labor at home with an inspired, independent midwife was far less painful than hospital births, which involved induction, epidural, laboring flat on my back, forceps, and emergency cesarean section. Subsequent births included a transfer to the hospital when I had been booked for home and I know all about how painful it can be when the baby is malpositioned – although I also know the triumph of overcoming it without medical assistance.

I managed my last three labors with the help of **a** TENS machine (see pages 111–113). I am very proud of having introduced these to the pregnant public in 1984, with the generous help of Roy Sherlock of Neen Healthcare who was responsible for importing them from Sweden. At that time, they had only been used in hospital trials during the 1970s, and could only be used under a doctor's supervision. Enabling women to use one at home in early labor gave back some of the control removed by hospital birth, and their popularity proves how welcome they have been.

When I started writing this book I hoped to discover some well-guarded secret that would ensure that you didn't have to experience labor as painful. Many people have passed on helpful hints, but I have come to the conclusion that there is no magic bullet.

And that is the point: giving birth is all about growing up and taking responsibility for yourself and your baby. It is a big step, and may not be easy. The truth that does emerge, though, is that at heart you do know what is best for you and what will help you most.

Listen to your subconscious and don't allow it to be overruled. Trust your instinct; it won't let you down.

Chapter One

THE PROCESS OF LABOR

"How and when will labor start?" "Will I know when I am in labor?"

These questions can recur repeatedly in the minds of pregnant women – particularly those expecting their first baby. Although this is partly due to the self-absorption of pregnancy, and it can be fun to envisage various different scenarios, they are questions that can become worrying. And while some people relish the uncertainty and potential drama, others would very much like to know the answers. For most people, the timing of labor is unpredictable, and even when predictions are made they are not reliable. But it is a matter of absorbing interest; every twinge and sign may be examined minutely. Although it is rare, but not impossible, to be well advanced in labor without realizing it, the reverse is much more likely; when you have a spell of contractions; a touch of diarrhea or even a "show," you may be convinced (or may want to be) that this is it, when actually it isn't. In fact, labor can be a lengthy limbering-up process with apparent stops and starts, rather than the dramatic sudden groan and imperative dash to the hospital beloved of dramatists.

Every labor starts differently, although women with more than one child may be able to detect a trend that is individual to them. In some cases it will become clear in retrospect; for example, if you have a backache, apparently unrelated to contractions.

· *When Will the Baby Arrive?* ·

Some inconsistencies are produced by attempts to make exact reckoning for pregnant women: for when the time fixed for their delivery is past the mistake creates much solicitude and impatience, when therefore it is necessary to give an opinion on this subject it is better to mention some time beyond that which we really suppose for on the whole it would perhaps be better that labor should always come on unexpectedly.

Thomas Denman
Introduction to the *Practise of Midwifery*
London, 1782

Little has changed since 1782, although the introduction of ultrasound has supposedly taken the guesswork out of pregnancy dating. Even when there is no doubt over the timing of conception – as with in vitro fertilization (IVF) – the length of pregnancy will naturally vary between mothers.

Surveys have shown that there is a five-week period in which labor may start "normally" (Mittendorf 1990, Saunders 1991). The belief that pregnancy lasts for ten menstrual cycles, or 40 weeks from the start of the last period, is based on Naegele's rule, unchanged since the 1800s, and not based on research. It is a convenient figure, but disregards the fact that 70 percent of women go into labor after their estimated date of delivery. Three percent of babies arrive on their due date.

Individual characteristics can make a difference. Women with several children may notice a trend particular to them: they may always go into labor early or late.

Mittendorf found that women under nineteen or older than thirty-four, those who were black, or for whom it was not a first baby, were statistically more likely to go into labor before others. He also found that height made a difference: the taller a woman was, the longer pregnancy was likely to last. The average length of pregnancy for white women expecting their first baby was 41 weeks and one day.

Ultrasound measurements can be inaccurate, for the obvious reason that babies are of different sizes at any given age – just as their weight can vary widely at birth. At 16 weeks gestation a fetus whose biparietal diameter (measurement across the head) measures 1 SD (spectral doppler) above the standard is equal to one who measures I SD below average at 18 weeks. One SD covers two-thirds of the population – so allowing a 14-day margin of error.

A woman with a regular menstrual cycle generally ovulates 14 days before her period: day 14 in a 28-day cycle, day 21 in a 35-day cycle, etc. If you had a positive pregnancy test shortly after missing a period your dates will be as accurate as those by ultrasound. If you know when you conceived, you should refuse to be budged by ultrasound estimates.

A good rule for everyone might be Montgomery's Rule, an observation that he made in 1837:

"a very common calculation among women themselves is to reckon 42 weeks from the last menstruation or 40 weeks from the middle day of the interval."

· *Oxytocin and Pitocin* ·

Oxytocin is the naturally occurring hormone, present in the bodies of both men and women, particularly involved in the process of reproduction. It is produced in the hypothalamic region of the brain and secreted by the posterior pituitary gland. It plays a part in conception (Robertson 1994) by playing a part in the manufacture of sperm, by causing contractions of the uterus following orgasm which help to suck sperm into it and by increasing the mobility of the fallopian tubes thus aiding the transport of sperm up the tubes.

Oxytocin helps to maintain the pregnancy by contracting the uterus at intervals to help keep the cervix closed. Labor starts when estrogen and progesterone balances change, which results in an increase of natural prostaglandin in the body. This results in a change in reaction to the effect of oxytocin in the area of the cervix, when it begins to soften and open rather than remaining tightly shut as it has been throughout normal pregnancy.

As pressure from the baby's head is exerted against the cervix, oxytocin is released, resulting in contractions. While membranes are still intact the pressure from the presenting part – usually the head – will exert sufficient pressure to encourage contractions that are manageable. If the membranes rupture either naturally or are artificially ruptured, the pressure on the cervix and resultant increase in the outpouring of oxytocin can make contractions suddenly much stronger and more intense. Oxytocin production can be inhibited (see page 31) by the release of adrenaline if a woman feels apprehensive about the situation in which she is laboring.

Oxytocin in increasing amounts carries the labor through to the second stage with a further surge as the baby's head opens out the pelvic floor muscles and a final surge as the head touches the perineum. This provides enough oxytocin to push the baby out and ensure that colostrum is present in the breasts for the baby immediately after birth.

Oxytocin helps the contractions to continue after birth to expel the placenta and is responsible for the production of breast milk and the all important milk-ejection or let-down reflex that causes milk to flow in response to the baby's suckling.

· *Indications That Labor May Be Starting* ·

It is clear that with the start of labor, as with the rest of labor, the mind can play a part. For example, women may wait until they know a midwife they particularly like is on duty, or labor at night if they are having their baby at home and already have children. It is striking how many people go into labor spontaneously when in the hospital and booked for induction the following morning.

Weight Loss
There may be a reduction in the amount of amniotic fluid surrounding your baby at the end of pregnancy which may mean that you stop gaining weight or start to lose it. You may lose as much as $2\frac{1}{4}$ pounds in the last few days before labor starts. You may also be able to feel the baby's outline more clearly.

Decrease in Movements
The baby becomes less active as labor approaches. If you are concerned about a decrease in movements you should ask your midwife to check the baby's heart

Nesting Instinct
Some women, not all, experience a sudden burst of energy and feel driven to clean or clear up. An urge to clean the oven is pretty diagnostic. Try to conserve energy to some extent: you may need the energy for labor.

Diarrhea or Stomach Upset
Hormone changes prior to labor can result in frequent bouts of diarrhea or a feeling of stomach cramps similar to stomach upset. Diarrhea has the advantage of clearing the bowel so that its contents do not impede the baby's progress.

Feeling Irritable
Some women feel particularly irritable prior to the start of labor and can be uncharacteristically snappy. Some may feel "different" or actually unwell. Others may feel especially well.

Show
The show is the mucus plug that fills the cervix during pregnancy and acts as a barrier between the cervical opening into the vagina and the baby and bag of membranes. As the cervix alters shape at the very start of labor, the plug becomes free and drops out. The plug can vary quite widely in appearance: it may be a clear, solid, jellylike, thimble-sized

lump, or it can be quite runny and bloody. If you bleed enough to soak a pad you should contact your midwife or doctor, in case it is a sign that the placenta is becoming detached.

If the plug has come away spontaneously, labor should start within thirty-six hours, although it may be longer. It can come away prematurely if you are checking your cervix yourself, are given a "sweep" of the membranes, or make love.

Contractions

You will probably have started to become aware of the Braxton-Hicks contractions of the uterus from about 20 weeks of pregnancy onwards, although some people seem to feel them less than others. This is when the uterus seems to swell and become hard and tight, lasting for about a minute, every fifteen minutes or so; perhaps more often if you are exercising. As pregnancy progresses, these contractions, which are designed to ensure that fresh blood reaches the uterus, become more noticeable.

When a set of Braxton-Hicks contractions occurs more frequently and lasts longer and is stronger than usual you may feel it heralds the start of labor. They can in fact become contractions that start to dilate the cervix – but may also last for as much as four hours before returning to normal. They may be more frequent if you remain in one position – for example, sitting or driving a car – as the uterus has to make more effort to circulate the blood. To see if it really is labor, try changing position. In the past it was said that true labor could be distinguished from these practice contractions by putting hot cloths onto the abdomen: contractions would either cease or become true labor.

Even if contractions do not continue they may still have been effective in starting to prepare your cervix by making it shorter, softer and thinner.

If contractions like these keep you awake, it may be worth taking acetaminophen with a hot drink on the grounds that you will need some sleep if it is going to be labor, and otherwise is not worth losing sleep over. There is no chance that you will sleep through labor, although the excitement of thinking it could be may keep you awake.

The contractions of labor become increasingly frequent, last longer, and are stronger in intensity. The textbook pattern is for them to come at say half-hour intervals, moving to twenty-five minutes, twenty minutes, fifteen minutes, ten minutes, etc., and then more often so at the end they last for longer than a minute and there may seem to be little breaks between them. There are variations on this theme – they may start at more frequent intervals and be every five minutes almost to the end, but they do increase in intensity. They may start by feeling like period pains or you may have a low backache that coincides with contractions. Some people get pains down their thighs; in some people the backache moves around to the front to become low abdominal pain.

If you are using a TENS machine it is best to put it on as soon as you are reasonably sure that you are in labor.

Rupture of Membranes

This occurs at the start of labor in about 10 to 15 percent of women, and is one of the things that people get concerned about. It mostly happens at night in bed, but if it does occur when you are out, it will be quite apparent that you are pregnant and no one will think that you have lost control of your bladder.

The amniotic fluid – generally known as the waters – can go in a rush or a trickle depending on the position of the baby, and the site of the membrane rupture. There may be an audible ping or pop and you may feel that something has "gone." You may just feel a bit damp or be drenched by a pint of warm liquid.

Amniotic fluid (known in the past as "silver water") is clear normally, and can have an individual smell that you may be able to identify even if you are not familiar with it. There can be confusion over whether liquid is urine or amniotic fluid; if you put on a pad and wait, it should become clear. Waters will continue to trickle and the flow will increase with Braxton-Hicks contractions. Amniotic fluid can be identified with reagent strips because it is alkaline; midwives keep swabs known as Amnistix that change color when they are in contact with amniotic fluid.

In most cases, contractions will start within a few hours of membranes rupturing (see page 35) and there is no urgency to do anything. However, there are some situations when you should get help:

- If your membranes rupture, or you think they may have, and you are not yet 36 weeks pregnant, you should go to a maternity unit immediately. Premature labor can start quite rapidly, although you will probably be encouraged to rest in the hope that the membranes will heal over. This will need to be in the hospital.
- If the amniotic fluid is colored, you should contact your midwife or doctor. This shows that the baby has passed meconium, the contents of its bowel, and may be a sign of distress. A golden

color indicates that it was passed some time ago so the distress is not current. A greeny-black color is fresh and means the baby should be checked right away.

- You should also contact a midwife or doctor if your membranes have ruptured and the baby's head is not engaged, that is, well into your pelvis. This may have been described as the head being high, or perhaps another presentation such as breech or transverse. If the head is not blocking the pelvis there is a slight risk (one in 400) that the cord could come out in front of the baby. This is rare and most commonly occurs following artificial rupture of the membranes, but is potentially life-threatening for the baby, because the cord can become pinched between the pelvis and the baby's head, cutting off its blood and oxygen supply.

    If your membranes rupture and you know or suspect that the baby's head is high or is not head down at all, lie down and get someone to call a doctor or midwife to come and check or get someone familiar with the baby's heartbeat to listen to it; cord compression will make it irregular. If there is any irregularity, or if you can feel the cord protruding or in your vagina, call an ambulance immediately and lie face down with your knees on the ground and your bottom in the air. Do not touch the cord, except to put it back into the vagina.

    Most women (70 percent) will go into labor and deliver within 24 hours of membrane rupture (Enkin 1990) and nearly all (90 percent) will deliver within forty-eight hours without any intervention.

Obstetricians are often concerned that ruptured membranes mean that the baby is no longer protected from infection within the vagina and like to induce labor in the absence of spontaneous contractions. However, evidence shows that inducing labor can reduce the time from membrane rupture to birth – thirty hours down to twenty-four on average – but labor lasted fifteen hours in the induced group compared with six hours in the group that was allowed to go into labor spontaneously. One trial of 900 women (Marshall 1993) found that allowing women to go into labor naturally meant that they had one-third as many cesarean sections as the group who had labor started artificially, and there was no increase in infection in the mothers or the babies.

If your membranes rupture when your pregnancy is full term, there seems to be a lot to be gained by waiting and letting nature take its course, although some obstetricians are still reluctant to "allow" this.

It makes sense not to increase the risk of intrauterine infection by not allowing vaginal examinations of any kind, not having sex, showering rather than bathing, and possibly taking eight garlic capsules and a gram of vitamin C every few hours to help prevent infection. You may want to compromise by taking prophylactic antibiotics if contractions have not started within forty-eight hours although it is debatable as to how effective this is.

It seems to be safe to have a bath or to labor in water once contractions have started (Eriksson 1996).

Feel of the Cervix

If you are able to reach your cervix, you will be able to make your own assessment about whether labor has started. If you are familiar with the way it feels normally, you will easily notice any change. As labor approaches, the tissues of the perineum, vagina, and cervix become noticeably softer. There may also be a marked increase in the flow of clear vaginal mucus.

If you want to check your cervix yourself, you or your partner should wash your hands thoroughly before making a gentle examination. It may be easier to do this sitting on the toilet or while standing with one foot resting on a chair. Insert two fingers and feel for the cervix which feels like a knob at the top of the vagina. If it is "unripe", or not ready for labor, it will be long, hard, thick, and closed and its shape will not have altered. When it is ready for labor it will have changed to feel softer, shorter, and thinner and it will have opened so that your fingertip fits in the opening. Your cervix can be "ripe" several weeks before the start of labor.

If you think that labor has started, you may want to feel your cervix to make sure. If it is high or out of reach, you are unlikely to be in labor because it becomes lower and more accessible as it dilates. If you can reach it, its edges may feel frayed or serrated and it will be very mobile. If you can feel the "os" or opening, you may be able to get two fingers inside it, particularly if this is not your first baby.

Once you are in established labor the baby's head moves down and you will be able to feel that it is lower. You may feel the cervix over the head. It may feel like something slimy over a grapefruit; it becomes paper-thin and very smooth. By this time it can be hard to get your fingers inside it because it will have changed shape from being a canal to being flat, fitting closely over the baby's head. The hole created by the dilating cervix is completely round, and when it is fully dilated 10 cm there is no rim of cervix left to be felt.

Repeated vaginal examinations are not recommended although there is a big difference between doing them yourself at home where your germs are your own and you will not hurt yourself, and having them done in a hospital environment. It can be fascinating to feel the waters behind the membranes and to touch your baby's head for the first time.

· *Early Labor* ·

Early labor can be a very exciting time. Contractions are tolerable, even enjoyable, and will not last all that long—and it can feel wonderful to know that you have reached the point that you have been waiting for and speculating about for so long. You will react differently depending on whether it starts in the day or night. If it is night-time, it really is better, if not always possible, to get as much sleep as you can. Rest as long as you can manage: fatigue makes it harder to cope in labor and can lead you to accept forms of pain relief that you would really prefer to do without. Some women find it easy to doze between contractions while others do not. Some acetaminophen, a hot drink and hot water bottle may help. If you can manage to play the whole thing down to start with it may not seem so long.

If labor starts in the day, carry on as normal. Women who already have children have plenty to keep them busy until contractions can no longer be ignored, but first-time parents may want to go shopping, swimming, or finish decorating. For some reason, couples often visit garden centers in early labor.

The hospital is a very limiting environment. Although you may be able to walk around the ward, or even outside, there is little to distract you compared with the number of things that you can find to do at home.

It is a good idea to eat and drink well in the early stages (see pages 72–75). There will come a point when your digestion shuts down and you may not feel like eating, or you may even be sick, but stocking up in the early stages will give you energy and reduce the risk of becoming dehydrated.

In the early first stage, pain may be felt around the lower abdomen, going around to the back. Later in first stage, it can reach further up the abdomen, up the back to waist height and low down over the hips. In the early part of second stage, it may reach the very low back and perineum, and just before delivery it may be felt most intensely in the perineum and at the tops of the inner thighs.

It can be very difficult when having a first baby to know exactly what is happening, or to be able to estimate how advanced labor is, how much longer it is likely to last or how much more painful it can be. Even experienced midwives can be wrong about these things, so not surprisingly, it is particularly difficult if you have no experience of labor.

The ideal situation is to have a midwife who will visit you, check dilation, and leave, while remaining in contact. This may or may not be available to you – although it is worth enquiring. It is likely to be possible for women planning a home birth, or for those who have employed independent midwives.

Going to the Hospital

It has been said that, with a first baby, you almost cannot leave for the hospital too late, and many women on a maternity ward may have gone in before labor was truly "established": that is, 3 cm of cervical dilation. The question of whether labor is established or not can be a vexing one. You may have been having painful regular contractions for hours, but technically labor is only recorded from 3 cm dilation, which is why women often say things like: "Well, I thought it was twenty-seven hours, but they have got it down as twelve."

If you are trying to decide whether it is time to go in, the following is a guideline. You should call the hospital if in doubt and to let them know when you are on the way. The staff may encourage you and reassure you over the phone, but will probably suggest that you come in if you sound doubtful. It is far easier nowadays to go in just for assessment, and you may feel that it saves face if, before you leave, you haven't called all your nearest and dearest to say the baby is on its way.

A rough guide for when to go to hospital includes:
- If you are in labor before 36 weeks
- If you are bleeding – even if it is a very heavy show
- If your membranes have ruptured or the fluid is colored (see pages 4–5, 34)
- If you cannot cope, or are very frightened
- If contractions are every five minutes or more often and last longer than a minute, unless you feel you can cope as you are.

If the pain is continuous, and particularly if you have bleeding, call an ambulance, as this could be a sign that the placenta is peeling away prematurely.

Obviously, you will have to take into consideration your journey time, traffic conditions, etc. Try to remain confident even though you may be surprised by the intensity of the contractions, and remember that although pain is normally a sign that something is wrong, labor is different.

Take things slowly and lock up carefully. If you really think that things are happening very quickly, don't panic but call your midwife, or an ambulance. A midwife is the first choice; she will carry equipment to help you give birth at home if necessary and you can remain there afterward. Ambulance drivers are obliged to take you to the hospital – even if you give birth at home – and they will take you to the nearest one in an emergency, not necessarily to your preferred hospital. Once you have decided to leave home, and have made sure that you have everything with you, call the hospital to let them know that you are on your way.

Traveling by car while having contractions can be very uncomfortable. You may be most comfortable in the back seat on all fours. Make sure you have your TENS machine on if using one. Take a bucket lined with a plastic bag in case you are sick, and put towels underneath you in case your membranes rupture. The chance of giving birth on the way is tiny, particularly if it is a first baby. It does happen, but so rarely as to pass into local legend. If it does, the important thing is to keep the baby warm, next to your bare chest and well-covered. Clear any mucus out of its mouth with a finger – and continue to the hospital. Do not try to cut the cord. On arrival, park carefully. There will be contingency plans for women in advanced labor and special parking arrangements for partners.

When you reach the ward (there will be wheelchairs available for women who find it difficult to walk) you should be greeted by someone who has already looked at your notes. By this time contractions will be slowing your progress and there will be times when it is hard to talk. Midwives appreciate this and there is no hurry. (Of course if there is urgency you will be swiftly moved into a delivery room).

Your greeting should be welcoming and friendly, but in moving to the hospital you are changing your environment to one with which you are less familiar, and it is quite common for contractions to slow down or stop at this stage. They will start again when you feel comfortable in your surroundings and with your caregivers.

You will have your details checked against your notes, and then be assessed to see whether you are in labor and if so, how advanced labor is. You may feel that if you are less than 3 cm dilated, you would prefer to go home; it will be easy to return later.

If labor is further advanced or if you prefer to stay in, your baby's heart rate will be monitored (see pages 81–84), and you will have your blood pressure and temperature taken. Fortunately, the routine shave and enema have been abandoned, although you might choose to have an enema if you feel particularly constipated.

Some units admit women directly to the room where they will give birth; others have a ward for women in early labor and move them to a delivery room when labor is advanced. Either can be disconcerting: it may be off-putting to hear other women in labor, and if you are in your own room there is little to concentrate upon apart from yourself. You may be offered a midwife or a midwifery or medical student to be with you all the time, or just have a midwife coming in from time to time if the unit is busy. You will always have access to help via a bell or buzzer. You can ask to be left on your own with your partner if you would prefer, and you should be asked whether you are happy to have a student present. You can change your mind at any time.

You may be free to wander round the hospital at this point, which can be slightly more interesting and less isolating. Remember to continue to eat (if you feel like it) and drink. Don't forget to empty your bladder at least every hour.

Your midwife should have seen your birth plan by now (earlier if you have met her before) but it is worth telling her how you are hoping to handle your labor. Communication is vital, as it is easy to be overwhelmed by the situation and allow things to happen because it seems to be routine. Good midwives will always tell you what is going on, explain any suggested procedure, and get your consent first, but they are not all like this (Hunt, Kirkham). If you are aiming to get through with the minimum of pain relief from drugs, establish at the start that you welcome positive encouragement toward that end. If you feel very strongly that you are not going to see eye to eye, it is best to ask for a change of midwife right away (see pages 41–42). If you and the midwife have different philosophies, you will be happiest apart.

• *The First Stage of Labor* •

All being well, you will be able to settle in with support from your midwife and birth partner(s), and be ready to get on with labor. Pain-relieving drugs (see chapter 9) are likely to be on hand if you need them. It can be less easy to remain upright and change your position frequently when you are in a fairly small room with a bed in it. Most labor rooms are poorly designed for mobility in labor – you may need to be inventive with pillows, a bucket (page 77), or birth ball (page 81).

Contractions generally become painful with the increased intensity and as the cervix dilates. It is thought that the fact that pain messages travel repeatedly along nerve fibers contributes to the added awareness of pain, and any pain becomes wearing after a while, however well you are able to tolerate it to start with. At this point you may start to use some of your repertoire of coping or distraction techniques. (See pages 43–44.)

Pain is normal in childbirth. The increased strength and intensity of contractions that you may identify as sensation or experience as pain is a sign of progress, and each contraction is a step closer to holding your baby in your arms. An increase in power is a sign of progress. There is no injury in normal labor so that it is safe to stay with the sensation. This pain, unlike all other types, is not an indication that something is wrong, and fighting it by tensing – a natural reaction to normal pain – is counterproductive. If something is wrong you will know it instinctively and be able to recognize the fact – you will have a sense that things are not right. Tell your caregivers.

Try welcoming contractions, moving toward them, and relaxing into them. This may require concerted effort and you may need your supporters to remind you – they can help by putting hands quietly on your shoulders. The simple breathing technique of breathing *slowly,* in through your nose and out through your mouth, combined with conscious relaxation of your abdomen can be useful.

When you are in established labor you are likely to become more introverted and less inclined to talk. You will need to rest between contractions, and you may find yourself sinking toward the floor. At this stage labor can feel very tiring and relentless. Unless you are used to running a marathon or doing other demanding physical activity where you carry on beyond the point where your body is telling you to stop, you may not believe the demands that are being made on you. You can feel as if you are being pushed to the limit and beyond, and be incredulous that you cannot stop when you feel that you have had enough.

You will probably be dependent on other people to suggest moving, changing position, or having a bath, or massage. It can help to have written out a list of your personal coping strategies beforehand so that they can suggest them to you. It is not always easy to think of these yourself at this point.

· *Transition* ·

Towards the end of the first stage – perhaps between your cervix being 7 cm and fully dilated at 10 cm – you may experience some of the sensations of the phase known as transition. This can be a confusing time, mentally and physically. It may include an involuntary change in behavior – you may find yourself shivering, your legs may tremble, you could feel a cramp in your legs or buttocks, want to push before you are fully dilated, or be sick. Sometimes known as the swearing stage, this can be the part where women feel that they have simply had enough and cannot cope any longer. They can become very irritable, demand pain relief, or lose patience with everyone present. You can also feel very fearful or out of control, and may be afraid that you or your baby will not survive.

This may be the point where your membranes rupture spontaneously if they haven't already. There may be a large gush or only a little fluid. There may also be some fresh bleeding, which shows that you have reached second stage. The baby's head may be putting great pressure on you, giving an erroneous sensation of needing to empty your bowels urgently. It can feel large and round like a grapefruit.

Transition marks the change in the type of work that your uterus is doing, from contractions that pull up the neck of the uterus into its body and reduce the space available to the baby so that it is moved through the pelvis, to contractions that actively expel it, which are shorter, more frequent, and expulsive.

It can be helpful, if you suddenly feel out of control, to recognize that you have probably started transition and that means the end is not far away. Making a noise can help you through this stage. If you find yourself grunting in the middle of a contraction you will be close to being able to push your baby out.

· *The Second Stage of Labor* ·

When your cervix is fully dilated you are said to have reached the second stage of labor. You may not feel the urge to push immediately; there may be a quiet spell with no contractions to allow you to recover a little. If you have not had drugs and remain upright you should be able to push just when your body tells you to. The impulse to push can be overwhelming and very hard to resist. It is powered by a surge of oxytocin as the baby's head reaches the perineum (Ferguson's reflex).

If you have had an epidural or a managed labor, you may not feel the urge to push as the epidural can remove it altogether along with the sensation of contractions. In this case, midwives or doctors will probably wait until the head is very low before encouraging you to push, and perhaps also allow time for the epidural effect to wear off. If the pushing urge does not come naturally, you may need to be guided by your midwife or doctor over when to push and then have to make a conscious effort.

If you have to push deliberately you may be urged to bear down with your chin on your chest, exerting pressure from your diaphragm downwards. It is thought to be better to give several short pushes rather than one long one because you invariably hold your breath to push effectively. Holding your breath for a long time can raise the pressure in your chest which prevents blood from returning to your heart. This results in falling blood pressure, a fall in the output of the heart, and a disruption of blood flow to the uterus and baby. Remind yourself that you have to help the baby slide down and round the curve of the birth canal and out through the vagina (some childbirth educators liken this to the curve of a banana or the movement necessary to put your foot into a tall boot).

If you and the baby are well, you may want to delay pushing until you do feel an urge. Artificial time limits on second-stage length may be enforced in the hospital. These are often two hours with a first baby and half an hour for subsequent children. Clearly there is no point in continuing to push a baby out if it is irrevocably stuck in the pelvis or too big to get through, but pelvic ligaments stretch during the second stage and the bones of the baby's head are able to overlap, both of which help to alter dimensions so that the baby can get through eventually. Pushing with a groan rather than a closed glottis (completely held breath) on the outward breath is a technique used in physical exertion by people during weightlifting or in the gym, and is the way women often choose when working instinctively with the expulsive contractions.

You will probably find that there is a position which seems right for the second stage – and you should trust your instinct, providing that there is someone ready to catch the baby. Your supporters may have to assist you to change position as moving can be very difficult at this point. You may find it is not the position that you anticipated or prepared for, but you will probably adopt the right position to help the baby maneuver its way through.

The pushing phase can be as short as two contractions or last for several hours. It can be exhausting, particularly if you are having to try to push, and it can be disheartening when it seems as though the baby keeps slipping back again. Progress may be slow but if it moves down and then back up again it will still be coming down a little bit more with each push.

Some women find the second stage very painful and others not at all. Most experience a splitting, bursting, burning sensation at the moment of crowning. It is important to relax the muscles of your pelvic floor consciously at this point in order to let the baby out. You should listen to instructions about not pushing; you may be told to pant. Although it can be tempting to give one almighty push, you stand a better chance of keeping your perineum intact by allowing the baby to ease its way out. You can put your hand down to protect your perineum and feel the baby's head.

Once the head is born the rest of the body follows easily. The baby will probably be a deep, blue-purple until it takes its first breath, after which it will turn pink. A new baby can be surprisingly messy: its skin may look water-logged or be covered in vernix, the waterproof cream that protects it from the amniotic fluid until it is due to be born. It can be streaked with blood and mucus and will have a thick white and blue cord coming from the area of the navel. He or she will have enlarged genitals and the head may be molded into a most peculiar shape by the passage through the pelvis (midwives can tell the position a baby was in during labor by the shape of the molding of the head). Unless you are familiar with newborn babies, you will probably find that it is very different from the way you imagined it.

Once your baby is born it may need mucus removed from its mouth or nasal passages, which may be done routinely in some places. The baby will then be given to you to hold and suckle.

• *Delivering the Placenta* •

Following normal labor, your emotion and the stimulus provided by the baby's suckling will release more oxytocin from your pituitary gland into the bloodstream. This stimulates further contractions of the uterus, so that it becomes smaller. The placenta will no longer be able to remain attached to the shrunken wall of the uterus and so it peels away. Subsequent contractions should ensure that it is delivered shortly after the baby. If the uterus does not contract or the placenta does not come away or it only partially detaches there is a risk of serious bleeding or postpartum hemorrhage.

It is to reduce this risk that an injection of Pitocin or Syntocinon (synthetic oxytocin) may be given routinely as the baby's shoulders are born. This ensures that the uterus will contract down hard within seven minutes. The placenta has to be delivered beforehand or it will be trapped within the uterus. It also means that the umbilical cord has to be clamped before the strong, artificially stimulated contractions force extra, unnecessary blood into the baby. Staff may have to pull on the cord in order to get the placenta out in time. If it fails to come out, then either you have to wait for the effects of the Pitocin to wear off, or the placenta has to be removed manually under general anaesthetic. Some women find that Pitocin makes them feel sick.

The complex issue of receiving synthetic oxytocin and its effects on the baby are discussed in Sally Inch's book, *Birthrights*. It seems that the third stage of labor will take place naturally and without the aid of an injection if you have had a normal spontaneous labor of average length. The placenta can take at least an hour to come away spontaneously, and there seems to be no harm in waiting if you are not bleeding heavily. The oxygen available to the baby via the blood in the cord before it stops pulsating naturally can be of value, especially if the baby is slow to breathe.

If you do bleed during a natural third stage you can be given an intravenous injection of Pitocin or Ergotrate that will work within forty-five seconds to contract the uterus.

Midwives are more open to withholding Pitocin these days, but it is a matter for discussion both before labor – and during it – if things are not going according to plan. In the case of sudden hemorrhage, it will not be open to debate.

Chapter Two

PAIN

Giving birth is an individual experience complicated by a vast range of factors, some of which are controllable, and many of which are not. Because it is not only a physical experience and because the implications of becoming responsible for a new life are so great, the range of feelings that are involved during the process is colossal. Labor pain – unlike other pain – is productive. However, despite being the most positive pain possible it can also be the most intense. Indeed, it has been rated as the most intense pain of all: thought to be worse than that felt by sufferers from back pains, cancer pain, phantom limb pain, shingles, toothache, and arthritis. There is no doubt at all that labor can be excruciating.

But the pain of childbirth is a complex issue. Normally, people in severe pain are offered and accept medication to help relieve the pain; there is nothing to lose and little to be gained by not having it. Labor, though, is different. Women may indeed be offered pain relief but they may not want to take it, feeling that they would prefer support and reassurance, or they are apprehensive about the effects on the baby, or even because they feel that labor pain is natural and so they should be able to tolerate it. Relatively pain-free labor has not been shown to increase women's satisfaction with the experience (Morgan 1982), although until it was available in the form of the epidural it was thought it would be welcomed wholeheartedly.

Labor pain differs from other types of pain, too, in that it increases gradually, it is intermittent, and the breaks are largely pain free. In the early stages it can be quite bearable, and even enjoyable, and although it can be intense and severe during the later stages, there are still brief breaks and you know that it will be over within 48 hours.

• Studies of Pain •

Ronald Melzack, a well-known specialist on the subject of pain, studied 141 women in labor to ascertain the level of pain that they were feeling. He found that it is among one of the severest pains that he had recorded, but the intensity ranged from mild to excruciating. It is important to remember that the pain is not severe throughout. It increases with dilation of the cervix and is most likely to be painful when contractions are coming frequently and lasting longer.

In his study, nine percent of first-time mothers and twenty-four percent of women for whom it was not a first baby had low levels of pain. You will get some idea of how women feel labor pain from the stories in this book. Melzack found that women described their pain in strikingly similar ways when offered an extensive list of descriptive words to choose from (The McGill Pain Questionnaire). Starting with the most frequently used description, sharp, which 62 percent of women used – it was felt to be cramping, aching, throbbing, stabbing, hot, shooting, and heavy. They also found it tiring (49 percent) and exhausting (36 percent), intense (52 percent) and tight (44 percent).

It is always hard to imagine pain and descriptions of labor pain may mean little until you experience them yourself. However, you may find it helpful to know of some of the ways that women describe it at the time, which include: burning, grinding, stony, overwhelming, worse than kidney stones, terrific, aching, bruising, back-breaking, as if about to pop, unable to move, like a screwdriver up the bottom, knifelike, as if my body was being invaded, the baby is in charge, powerful, relentless, intense, crampy, like period pain, like thunderbolts in the pelvis and vagina, excruciating, frightening, and purposeful.

Although Melzack recorded intense levels of pain at some point in labor for the majority of women, only 25 percent of first-time mothers and 11 percent of those who were already mothers rated it as horrible or excruciating – the top of the pain-scale range.

Clearly, some women feel more pain than others in a particular labor. There has been considerable interest in trying to determine whether various factors mean that it is possible to predict how painful individual women will find labor. It is clear that women who have good labor support and who feel comfortable in their environment – especially at home – require less pain relief. Other factors have been identified; as with almost all research, there is not necessarily a consensus, but the following categories of women have been found to be more likely to find labor painful: those who have had difficulty in accepting the pregnancy and experienced conflict over becoming a mother; those who had previously had psychological counseling or psychiatric treatment; those who felt particularly anxious about labor and who feared helplessness, pain, loss of control and loss of self-esteem. (Lederman 1979).

Other researchers, who looked at mainly physical factors, found that labor pains were more intense among those who were first-time mothers, younger, had had less education, more menstrual problems, a history of abortion (miscarriage and therapeutic), unstable emotional feelings, unrealistic expectations of pain and discomfort, more pain-relieving drugs during labor and delivery, and a mate with negative or indifferent feelings toward the pregnancy.

Evidently, many of these factors cannot be altered, and although it has been said that it is best to skip the first labor and go straight on to the second, it can't be done.

The two main areas that *can* be changed are feelings of anxiety prior to the birth, and unrealistic expectations.

• *Options and Expectations* •

Pregnancy allows plenty of time for research and the opportunity to prepare yourself. If you feel particularly apprehensive, you can use fear as a spur to find out ways of preparing yourself so that you are able to start labor feeling confident in your ability to cope, happy with the environment and your caregivers and supporters, but with a realistic appreciation of the pain that labor can cause, even when entirely normal and in ideal surroundings.

It is very important to find out about the options open to you and not just to accept what is offered, because you feel that "they know best". It is easy to believe that because this pregnancy is so important to you, everyone else regards it in the same way and is only working towards what is best for you. Pregnancy is a self-absorbing emotion – it has to be, to ensure that you constantly think of and protect your unborn child – but it can blind you to the fact that providers of maternity care have many other considerations as well. Midwifery and obstetric staff want the best for their clients but they also have considerations of staffing, costs, and other day-to-day concerns to think about.

General practitioners, for example, may have a loyalty to a particular unit, or refer you to an obstetrician whom they know rather than the best place for you. They may not be particularly interested in maternity care or continue to view the way that they learned to do things as the best – and they can be very opposed to home birth. Obstetricians may see birth primarily in terms of outcome: a healthy baby and a healthy mother. They may indeed know best, but in their terms, as they see it and in general, rather than as specifically applied to you.

You will not have that specialist knowledge, may never have seen someone in labor, and may not even be familiar with newborn babies and their needs or the needs of their mothers after birth. However, you are the expert on yourself and the only person who knows exactly how you are feeling and what your baby is doing now. You are the only one who can tell if any given proposal feels right or wrong to you and it is your instinct that you should trust. Although you can easily get the impression that it is the hospital that gets you the baby, it is you and your body which give birth.

Many women find that toward the end of pregnancy their views on where they want to have the baby have changed. This is not surprising: birth can seem very distant and unreal in the early stages, while the twinges of later pregnancy and the realization that the baby has to come out somehow can concentrate the mind powerfully.

However, late pregnancy is also often a time of comparative inertia. It is sometimes easier to think that you will settle for the place you are familiar with, that it's too late to change now, you'll do it for the next one, your partner is not sure about it, you will be able to handle it when you get there if you know what to say, etc. It does take effort to change. You may find it involves extra visits, negotiations, individual research – a chain of phone calls. If you are really not too bothered and think that you would feel the same about labor anywhere, then it may not be worth the effort. The process of giving birth does not seem to have the same significance for everyone: some women are mainly interested in the baby and not so concerned about labor.

If, however, you know that you have nagging doubts, you should act. Being aware that you were in a position to change things and failed to do so, for whatever reason, can be damaging to your self-esteem and your memory of your baby's birth – which you will never forget. Remember that you are acting for both yourself and your baby; you will be doing the best that you can for him or her too. If the baby's health is used to coerce you – "you don't want anything to happen to the baby" – analyze the argument carefully and accept any offer to show you the evidence.

Not everyone has a choice of maternity unit, although everyone can choose between hospital and home. If you feel you are unable to change your hospital, or it seems as though you are not getting the support from the midwives that you booked for home, then you need to make sure that the service you get is the one you want.

Maternity care providers are busy, their staff are often over-worked and under pressure, but now more than ever before they are geared to meeting women's needs. Of course they can only do this if they know what you want. It is pointless expecting them to do things the way you want them if you don't let them know what that is. This may seem like a statement of the obvious, but you can have such a clear idea about it that it can be hard to grasp that other people may have different views or experiences of doing it differently.

Communication must be a two-way process. Always be pleasant about what you want, acknowledge that there are different points of view but make it clear – politely – which way you want to do it. Do not be sidetracked or get angry; recognize that they are probably trying to do the best for you as they see it. You have more power than you may be aware of. Midwives are often under pressure from their hierarchy or from doctors and obstetricians. Your stated views give them authority to back you; your wishes are paramount except in the case of an emergency.

Being able to feel confident that you have done everything you can to find the right place to have your baby can be a great weight off your mind. If it was causing you concern you can feel as if a weight has lifted from your shoulders and find that it makes a substantial difference in the way you feel about your pregnancy: you will be able to relax into it and enjoy it more. Your baby will feel the release of tension.

• *Anxiety about Birth* •

If, however, you are happy about the place of birth but still feel very apprehensive about the birth itself, you need to tackle it. Some fear about the birth is normal. It is understandable that you should be concerned about an unknown experience, particularly one that is likely to be very painful. Some women particularly dislike the uncertainly of not knowing when it will be or how it will start, fear they will not know they are in labor, or that their waters will break in a public place. Perhaps more women dread an episiotomy and worry about wear and tear on their bodies – particularly that caused by obstetric intervention.

Prenatal classes

Prenatal classes are a great forum for discussing these concerns, giving you an arena in which to air your fears, making sure that you have an accurate idea of what might take place, and learning how to deal with whatever it is that is bothering you. They are well worth attending, particularly as they focus on the subject likely to be of greatest interest to you and to your fellow class members.

It can be wonderful to share pregnancy with other women at the same stage and be able to discuss how you are feeling and what is happening to you, knowing that other people can understand and sympathize. Friendships made there continue to be valuable as your babies start life – the minutiae of infancy which is all-important to you may not be of such interest to your friends without children – but those made prenatally will provide an invaluable sounding board for exchanging information, sharing feelings about broken nights, and providing your baby with a set of friends of his or her own age. Many prenatal group friendships continue as the children grow into their teens.

Prenatal classes vary depending on who is running them and they are often in great demand. Classes may be held at the hospital and may also be offered privately in your community.

Some prospective parents attend everything. This may not be necessary, although it can help to get an idea from the hospital or midwife about the way things are done at a particular unit, as well as an independent view. It also helps you to get to know people in your locality who are expecting babies – whom you will probably be meeting at the school door in five years' time. All classes should provide a forum for discussion, so that you can ask about alternatives, ask "what if . . ." questions and formulate an idea about what goes on. Class facilitators all have their own points of view, however objective they may try to be, so keep an open mind over what they say.

All prenatal classes aim to prepare you for labor as well as parenthood and will involve teaching you ways of enabling you to

consciously relax your body in response to contractions. Some
classes deal with it in more depth than others. Yoga classes can be
very good if you are interested in helping yourself in this way,
while the amount of relaxation taught in other classes depends to
some extent on the facilitator.

The question of whether prenatal classes or prepared childbirth
actually reduces labor pain has been of interest to researchers and
the evidence suggests they do reduce the need for medication. Of
course it is not the only aim of classes, and in one way the question
is irrelevant. If you are the sort of person who always wants to find
out more about the sort of thing that is going to happen to you, you
will want to attend classes.

Other potential benefits include a decrease in the length of labor.
There was no agreement over this, but researchers found:

- lower levels of uterine dysfunction requiring artificial oxytocins
  to augment labor
- fewer cases of raised blood pressure
- less maternal illness and less use of antibiotics after birth
- more stable heart rate readings in babies during labor
- more involvement by partners
- more positive feelings about birth and giving birth among
  women attending
- less pain was felt during labor
- less frequent use of forceps at delivery
- greater awareness at birth
- more enjoyment of birth for women who had attended classes
  than for those who had not.

• *Karen Heywood* •

*I'm from Zimbabwe where medicine is private and lots of women
have cesarean sections. Because I am just over five feet tall, a lot
of my friends from home assumed that that is what I would have
and were surprised that I was not scheduled for one.*

*In fact, I hadn't thought a great deal about labor until we
attended prenatal classes. When I did, I found that the idea of
natural childbirth appealed to me and I was tempted to plan a
home birth. The problem was that we had recently moved so
that it did not feel like home, and my parents would be staying
and they might have found it more stressful than us. However*

*I didn't feel positive about the hospital and didn't really want
to give birth there.*

*Labor started with some false alarms. I went into the
hospital on Thursday night because I felt that I was having
contractions and some of the symptoms that we had talked
about in class. They said that my cervix was softening but not
dilated. It happened again the following night but by Saturday
morning the contractions had stopped again. They started
again later but did not get closer together, so I labored at
home, leaning over a beanbag and practicing relaxation
techniques.*

*We went into the hospital at 11 P.M. on Saturday and
found that I was 4 cm dilated. By 2 A.M. I was not much further
on, despite having a lot of contractions. They eventually
suggested rupturing my membranes artificially and warned
that it might come hard and fast after that. I had not wanted
this but I was quite worried because I had been in labor a long
time and I was very tired, so I agreed. The head was still not
engaged and although I kept breathing through the contractions
and found it helpful to squat on a small stool, I got very tired.
The midwife suggested Demerol but I asked for and got a
milder narcotic. By around 7 A.M. I was 6 cm. After that
medical things kept being suggested. I found it very useful that
previous discussion in class meant that I knew what they were.*

*After lunch they suggested Pitocin and an epidural
because the head was still not engaged. I think it was in a bad
position. I agreed to this but having the epidural was the worst
thing about it all. The doctor who was doing it took a long time
and bumbled about; by this time I was in transition and got
very panicky. I found it very hard to keep still in one position
and yet was frightened to move because it was so close to my
spine. I felt like a slab of meat. The obstetrician came around
and put the epidural in again so that I was more comfortable.*

*Up until then I had felt involved but then I found that
things did not go the way that I would have chosen. I ended up
on my back, although when we talked in class it had seemed to
make so much sense to be upright. There were a student
midwife and a student doctor there which made me feel
overwhelmed and less able to ask for what I wanted, and of
course I was very tired. I did manage to get them to get me
leaning forward over pillows – it was easier to push like that –
but although there was a tremendous feeling of pressure and I*

was pushing and pushing, I couldn't feel anything happening.

The doctor came and looked at the monitor and said the baby was in some distress, although they managed to calm me and say that on the whole it was OK. I kept looking at the monitor to see if it was all right. Eventually they decided it would have to be a cesarean: they did try to adjust her position but it didn't work.

Patrick found it all stressful too, although it made an enormous difference to have him with me all the way through. The staff were very sensitive to the fact that this was not what I would have chosen and did their best in a very stressful situation. I didn't feel that anything they did was for their convenience and they made a final check before they actually did the operation. Georgina was fine when she was born but clearly angry. She weighed 6 pounds 12 ounces so was not huge.

I think the whole experience would have been a lot more frightening if we had not been to prenatal classes.

Expectations

Women's expectations of birth have been examined in detail too. This is an interesting area because by and large women with positive expectations of labor have a positive experience and vice versa (Slade 1993, Crowe 1989, Green 1993). This seems contradictory in a way: it might appear at first that women with a negative view are merely being realistic about the degree of pain they are likely to experience. However, the key factor seems to be the degree of anxiety that the prospect of giving birth causes. Several studies (Newton C 1991, Stolle 1987, Fridh 1990, Morgan 1990) have shown that women did not anticipate the level of pain that they actually experienced. Newton found that almost half thought the pain was much worse than expected. This can work both ways: women who had already had one child anticipated that the pain levels would be similar in a second birth, but actually overestimated their need for pain relief (Fridh 1990).

If you are realistic about the likely degree of pain – which is hard, because it is not easy to imagine pain – does it not follow that it must cause you anxiety? Logically speaking it must: there can be few pregnant women who have not felt a twinge of panic at the thought of giving birth, even if they have done it before. Experienced mothers often suddenly remember previous labor with clarity at about 38 weeks gestation. However, feeling nervous and using those nerves to prepare yourself for birth as best you can, and feeling deep anxiety, are different matters. You will know yourself if you tend to be anxious, or if you are normally sanguine but are very concerned about the prospect of labor.

Dealing with Fear
Studies have found that 20 percent of women suffer from fear of delivery and that for 6 percent, the fear is incapacitating. As we have seen, anxiety about labor can create a self-fulfilling prophecy because it increases the stress and tension felt and makes labor longer and more painful. Interestingly, a Swedish study showed that it was not pain that caused women most anxiety (44 percent), or fear of death of themselves or their babies (55 percent), or their inadequacy physically or mentally to give birth (65 percent), but lack of trust in obstetric staff during delivery (73 percent).

If you feel that anxiety is spoiling your pregnancy it is important to seek some help as soon as possible. If you suffer from anxiety normally, see your general practitioner about getting some psychological support. If your anxiety is related purely to pregnancy, it may be best to get help through your maternity caregiver. In either case, it is important to talk about it and to take the other steps, such as prenatal classes or hypnotherapy, in order to prepare yourself.

Chapter Three

PHYSIOLOGY OF LABOR

From ancient times, until comparatively recently, it was believed that labor was initiated by the child and that the first stages of labor consisted of its attempts to make its way out of the womb. It knocks at the door asking to be let out. Kicking in the seventh month was believed to be a phase of preparing to leave, and the baby getting into the correct position. Only the second stage required the mother's efforts as well; she and her baby had to co-operate to allow birth to take place.

Nowadays, labor is known to be caused by powerful movement within the muscle of the uterus, although it is still not certain what initiates it.

The uterus has held the baby in, safely and well for the past nine months. In most cases, the sphincter at the cervix has been tight enough to keep the baby, placenta, and amniotic fluid within the uterus despite the combined pressure of weight and gravity. It is not surprising that opening the cervix (the neck of the uterus) sufficiently wide to allow a baby's head and body through, and the involuntary expulsive efforts required to push a baby weighing 8 pounds or more through the pelvis and the opened cervix are considerable.

Argument rages about whether this extraordinary process should be painful. The majority of women find it so, and many find it intensely painful, but the degree of pain experienced differs widely from woman to woman and from labor to labor with each mother.

Labor pain is physiological – there are distinct causes and the way the pain is registered in the brain is well recognized – but it is also psychological. It can be hard to credit the extent to which emotional or mental factors can influence the degree of pain felt, the length labor takes, and whether instrumental delivery becomes necessary.

Experienced midwives are familiar with the way in which the presence or absence of a particular person can speed or halt labor, and know how women can continue to labor and hold on to a baby until they reach an environment where they feel safe.

· *What is Pain?* ·

There are various definitions of pain, but it is caused by noxious sensory input to the central nervous system. Normally, pain is intended to cause a reflex action to move away from whatever is causing it, and to force us to recognize why we have it so that we can take action. Pain is normally associated with actual or potential tissue damage.

Pain receptors (nociceptors) are found in the skin, subcutaneous tissue, periosteum (the outer covering of bone), joints, muscles, and internal organs (viscera). Pain signals from any of these areas are transmitted via nerves to the spinal cord.

There are chemical and mechanical nociceptors in the ovaries, uterus, and broad ligaments. The uterus does not normally produce pain signals as it is insensitive to all sensations except those of twisting and stretching such as with labor or periods. However, it does contain chemical nociceptors, and repeated stimulation by contractions leads to production of substances that are produced in the body when tissue is damaged. These chemicals – bradykinin, histamine, serotonin, acetylcholine and potassium ions – are released into the bloodstream as a response to injury. Although they are part of the healing process they also cause pain.

· *Pain in Labor* ·

In the first stage of labor, pain messages from the uterus, cervix, and pelvic ligaments predominate. Pain sensations from these areas are transmitted through sympathetic nerves at vertebrae levels Thoracic 10 down to Lumbar 1 in the lower back. The TENS machine (see page 111) works partly on the principle of interfering with the transmission of these messages.

The dilation of the cervix is thought to give rise to much of the pain produced at this stage, unlike the Braxton-Hicks contractions of pregnancy which, although they may be as powerful as the contractions of early labor, are generally pain free.

As the baby moves downwards in the late first stage and early second stage, pain comes from distension and pulling on the pelvic structures surrounding the vagina. Eventually, pain results from the stretching of the perineum when pain messages are sent through the lower vertebrae, Sacral 2 to Sacral 4.

Throughout labor, pain signals may be sent as a result of the effect of pulling and pressure on internal organs, particularly the bladder, urethra and rectum, pressure on the spine exerted by the baby, and reflex muscle spasm in the spine. Referred pain is often felt in the abdomen, buttocks, hips, down the thighs and in the back. This is caused by pain from organs that is traveling along the same nerve pathways as that from sensory nerves, so that the messages can become confused and the brain interprets the pain signal as coming from an area other than the one which is actually sending it. Labor can also make skin hypersensitive.

Endorphins

The body is able to counteract these painful stimuli by producing its own natural opiates or painkillers called endorphins. Production of endorphins is a natural response to physical stress when a body is pushed beyond normal endurance. They create a feeling of well-being, modify pain, and can be responsible for change in awareness of time and space. They are the chemicals to which people who do a lot of physical exercise can become addicted because they make them feel so good, and are also responsible for the "second wind" that your body can produce when physically pushed. They are produced naturally during pregnancy. Levels gradually rise towards the end of pregnancy and can be responsible for feelings of well-being, readiness to have the baby, and particularly vivid dreams and periods of wakefulness at night. Endorphins can also have the effect of causing amnesia and so are responsible for the well-known forgetfulness of pregnant women – and also the way labor pain can be forgotten later. Provided their production is not blocked by reducing the sensation of physical stress as an epidural does, levels will rise until the baby is born.

Experience of Pain

Clearly, some people find labor pain more intense than others, although everyone is said to have the same sensory threshold. Pain levels will vary depending on whether it is a first or subsequent baby, the size of the baby, the position it is in, the time labor takes, and whether women have had previous experience of pain. Being familiar with pain can help to reduce the experience of pain in labor, unless the pain was caused by periods. Labor can be more painful in this case, because the body produces higher levels of prostaglandins which make contractions more intense.

Pain in labor alters during its course, but does not necessarily grow stronger all the time. It may wax and wane, although increased cervical dilation is associated with increased pain, particularly because contractions become more frequent, last longer and are stronger.

As a pain experience, labor is unique because it invokes so many different sensations and emotions and because it results in a very positive experience, the birth of a baby. The implications of going into labor are immense; life is about to change forever and a woman may feel excitement, apprehension, exhilaration, fear, and any combination of other emotions. Provided she feels confident in her ability to cope, and feels supported and safe, her body is free to produce endorphins to help her through labor.

Stress Hormones

However, if she becomes frightened and anxious – either because of the pain or because she does not feel comfortable with her surroundings or caregivers – her body will produce stress hormones, catecholamines, which can result in a vicious cycle of increasing the pain by reducing the blood flow to the uterus. Decreased blood flow to the uterus deprives it of oxygen and makes contracting more painful. In addition, the rise in adrenaline will act to reduce output of oxytocin – the hormone which is responsible for the maintenance of contractions – so that labor will slow or stop. Moreover, adrenaline has the effect of contracting the circular fibers in the lower third of the uterus to prevent further dilation. These muscles are then working in the opposite direction to the longitudinal and figure-of-eight muscle fibers in the uterus so that a painful tug-of-war ensues, resulting in painful apparent contractions but no further dilation of the cervix.

It is worth examining the effect of catecholamines in more detail because this natural response, which is simply the body reacting to a mother's feeling of unease about this being the right place to give birth, is responsible for a lot of current obstetric intervention.

While under stress of either a physiological or psychological nature, the body produces hormones including epinephrine (adrenaline) and norepinephrine (noradrenaline) and others. These hormones are responsible for the fright/fight/flight response with which we are familiar in response to an accident or threatening situations, and normally result in increased oxygen uptake, increased heart rate and blood pressure, elevated blood sugar, reduced peristalsis (squeezing movements of the intestines), shunting of blood from nonvital organs (including the uterus) to organs and skeletal muscles to prepare us either for flight or fight.

In labor, provided that the woman is not particularly anxious, catecholamine levels remain normal or lower than in pregnancy. As labor progresses catecholamine levels may increase in response to pain and consequent anxiety.

These catecholamines have a positive effect on the baby, which is also producing its own as a result of the stress of labor. This results in a drop of the baby's heart rate while under stress, which reduces its oxygen expenditure; blood is shunted from nonvital organs to the baby's brain, liver, and heart; the baby's ability to take up oxygen from the maternal blood is increased; and energy stores are mobilized. The baby, therefore, is able to cope with the reduction of oxygen supply during contractions, and is prepared for life after birth because of the effect of norepinephrine. This is the major hormone produced by the baby. It helps to promote absorption of liquid in the lungs, protects the heart and brain against lack of oxygen, and stimulates the ability to maintain body temperature. It also has the effect on the baby of making it appear wide-eyed, alert, and very warm at birth, which makes it appealing to the mother.

If a woman becomes very anxious, angry, upset, or tearful in labor she may produce excessive catecholamines which can decrease the efficiency of contractions by shunting the blood away from the uterus and placenta. As a result, the baby will get a reduced supply of oxygen. This may cause fetal distress, which will show in abnormal heart monitor readings and abnormal fetal blood pH samples. If stress continues in the mother, the baby may produce excessive catecholamines itself, which can cause problems such as breathing difficulties, jaundice, cold stress, acidosis, decreased plasma volume, and necrotizing enterocolitis after birth.

Most babies are healthy enough to withstand even excessive stress caused by the catecholamines produced by a woman who is unhappy about what is happening to her in labor. Babies who are fit at the start of labor will be able to withstand the pressure. However, it is obvious that if blood and oxygen are shunted away from the uterus it cannot perform as efficiently. Contractions will be diminished, labor will be prolonged, and the cycle of more anxiety and increased catecholamine output will repeat itself, leading eventually to labor "failing to progress" and possibly fetal distress.

There are two ways out of this dilemma. The first, which is commonly used, is to give the woman pain relief or sedation. This can help by breaking the cycle, although synthetic oxytocin may be given as well to stimulate contractions, perhaps before the pain relief can take effect. As catecholamine levels are reduced labor can accelerate. The medication crosses the placenta and depresses brain metabolism, reducing the baby's need for oxygen.

The other way, much less frequently used, is to reduce the stress so that the problem doesn't arise; ideally before labor, but otherwise by taking action once the problem has arisen during labor. It is worth looking at the things which increase and decrease stress in labor so that you can influence them to minimize the stress and pain you might feel. Not all these things are under your control but there are more than you may think. Preparing carefully can actually affect the nature of your labor.

• *Induction of Labor* •

Labor should only be induced if the risks of continuing the pregnancy outweigh the harm that may be done by starting labor artificially. However, this is rarely clear-cut and all sorts of other factors can affect the decision of a woman to accept or ask for induction, or to prompt medical staff to offer it.

Some of the reasons – which include the risk of physical harm to the mother or the baby – include preeclampsia, proven fetal growth retardation, Rhesus (Rh) incompatibility, maternal disease such as diabetes, and possibly postmaturity: the baby being overdue.

There are situations in which you will be in little doubt that the baby should be delivered soon, even though you may be very disappointed that you are not able to go into labor spontaneously. These could include such things as your having high blood pressure and it continuing to rise despite treatment, or you being aware that the baby is hardly moving.

However, over the issue of postmaturity in particular, medical opinions can differ widely from hospital to hospital and from obstetrician to obstetrician within the same hospital. If one doctor "likes to see the baby in the crib at 38 weeks" and another has "not induced a woman's labor for the past three years," then you can be sure that it is not women's individual needs which are being assessed when induction is recommended.

For the reasons discussed on page 2, 40 weeks is not the average length of pregnancy, although still regarded as such by many maternity staff, and by mothers who are led to believe that to be pregnant for longer means the baby is overdue. There are risks to the baby associated with going very much past 40 weeks because the baby is more likely to pass meconium into the amniotic fluid, with the risk of inhaling it at birth. However, this has to be balanced against the risks of induction.

Being given, or accepting that there is a date that the baby should arrive, can lead to real frustration when the day comes and goes and the baby shows no sign of arriving. The trouble is that you will have had this date in your mind for months, even when you know that it is only an approximation, and that the baby may quite normally be born at any point in a five-week period around that date – and it is more likely to be after it than before.

It is understandable that you can find days after the "due" date dragging and are impatient to see your baby. Moreover, if you cannot be relaxed about it – for example, if you have a limited amount of maternity leave, and people are constantly calling to find out if anything has happened, and if not, how long are "they" going to allow you – it can be easy to succumb to the invitation to "bring you in" on a certain day for induction. It is important to appreciate what is involved before agreeing, however, because induction of labor, particularly if you are not close to going into labor spontaneously, can have both long- and short-term repercussions for you and your baby.

Induction Procedures
Induction of labor always takes place in a hospital, although one of the procedures that is commonly used by midwives to encourage labor to start – that of sweeping or stripping of the membranes from the cervix – can be done at home.

Being in the hospital has the disadvantage that you will be there throughout labor with little to distract you. It is usual to be admitted the previous night. You will have your history checked and a vaginal examination when your cervix will be assessed to see how ripe it is; that is, how close you are to going into labor naturally. If it is soft and partially effaced you may be left until morning but if it is long and hard you will be given prostaglandin gel to soften it in preparation for induction. In some women, this is sufficient to start labor that night. Others, who have not been given the gel but are overdue, frequently start labor without it.

If you are not in labor, you will be given a light breakfast and will be admitted to the maternity ward. After further assessment gel will be inserted into your vagina, close to the cervix, and you will have to remain lying down for at least half an hour while it takes effect. If it starts contractions, this may be all you need. In some women it can provoke very intense and rapid labor. If not, you may be given further gel. If this does not start labor, you may also be offered artificial rupture of membranes and a Pitocin drip.

Artificial rupture of membranes or amniotomy (ARM) is done by having you lie on your back with your legs in stirrups while the doctor inserts an amnihook into your vagina and through the cervix. The amnihook looks like a long plastic crochet needle. When twisted, the hook on it nicks the membranes and the amniotic fluid gushes out. This is a painless procedure if the cervix is ripe; if not, it can be extremely painful.

These procedures, combined, should start labor. In fact they mean that the obstetrician is committed to delivering your baby within twenty-four to forty-eight hours by cesarean section, if necessary, because of the likelihood of having introduced bacteria from the vagina into your previously sterile uterus with consequent risk of infection to you or your baby.

If amniotomy fails to start your uterus contracting, you will be given synthetic oxytocin (Pitocin) intravenously, through a drip in the back of your hand. You may be offered an amniotomy and Pitocin at the same time which can make labor shorter, although there are risks associated with Pitocin.

One of the big disadvantages of having labor started artificially is the increased likelihood of requiring or being given other obstetric procedures – known as the "cascade of intervention". Clearly, there is a higher rate of cesarean section among women who have labor induced, but there is also an increased need for pain relief because contractions start off lasting longer and being stronger than in natural labor. There is a greater risk to the baby (Thornton 1994) as Pitocin-induced contractions can deprive it of oxygen for longer and the increased levels of analgesics can affect its behaviour after birth. There is a higher rate of forceps deliveries and vacuum extraction and more babies require special care after birth as a result of being short of oxygen at birth. Fewer women breastfeed following induced labor (Rajan 1994).

The experience of induction varies, depending on how rapidly your body responds to the stimuli. For some women with prolonged pregnancy it is relatively simple and easy. For others, particularly those whose cervices are not ripe, or who may not have gone into labor spontaneously for reasons connected with the baby's position, it can be a very long, drawn-out and unpleasant business, culminating in an operative delivery.

Agreeing to Induction

If induction of labor is recommended for you, it is likely to be prescribed as a matter of necessity and it can be difficult to disentangle the degree of need from the other factors involved. It can also be tempting to agree if you have no direct experience of labor and its aftermath, but it is essential to make sure that it really is warranted; that is, the risks to your health, or that of your baby are greater if you remain pregnant awaiting natural labor, than if it started artificially.

This means that you should be able to ask for and receive detailed information, including the results of fetal monitoring (see page 81–84) or other tests on your baby, as to why induction is considered necessary for you. If the answer relates to policy – "we only allow women to go ten days past their dates" – then you are entitled to refuse, perhaps compromising by having fetal monitoring at regular intervals.

Of course, no one can compel you to be induced, but the veiled threat "you wouldn't want anything to happen to your baby" is a powerful one and very hard to resist. Nearly every woman will put her baby's health first and accept induction if she is convinced it is for the best. If you are doubtful about it, ask around and get a second opinion. Midwives and clinic staff will be well aware of obstetricians' views, and can give you informal information on their views on induction and point you in the direction of the most liberal. If you have a trusting relationship with your midwife you can ask her what she would do in the circumstances.

Many midwives feel uneasy about routine induction, although they are not in a position to countermand it if you are under an obstetrician's care.

If you agree to induction, there are various points to bear in mind:

- Labor is likely to be more painful, although it may be shorter if Pitocin is given. You should be able to choose whether to have your membranes ruptured and await contractions, or to have Pitocin at the same time as the ARM.
- If you are not ready to go into labor, it may take a long time; if it fails to work you will have to have your baby delivered by cesarean section.
- Pitocin involves having a drip put into the back of your hand, which is uncomfortable. You will not be able to move around unless the drip is attached to a mobile stand.
- If you find the contractions are so painful that you need an epidural – and twice as many women have epidurals when labor

is induced – you are more likely to need an instrumental delivery – and twice as many women who have an epidural have an assisted delivery (Dept of Health 1997). An epidural can lead to a cycle of slowing labor so that more Pitocin is required.

You may feel that if labor has been so managed up until now, you may as well be plugged into everything. If that is your choice then that is fine, but if you find it upsetting to be induced and would much prefer to go into spontaneous labor, you may want to avoid an epidural. You will need support with this so ask for a midwife who is able and prepared to help you. It is possible to cope with induced labor without heavy pain relief, but it is harder. Stock up in advance with everything that you think will help – but most important, do not agree to it unless you are sure it is necessary.

Other Methods of Starting Labor
Induction is occasionally a matter of urgency but there is generally a period of time, often days, when it is under review and you have a chance to try other methods of starting labor. They include:

- **Sex**   Semen contains prostaglandin and can work in a similar way to prostaglandin gel, although it is less concentrated. Frequent sex, followed by lying on your back with a pillow under your bottom for at least half an hour, can start labor.
- **Nipple or breast stimulation**   Stimulate your nipples for 15 minutes or more several times a day, or gently massage your breasts for three hours a day spread over two to three sessions. This has been shown to increase cervical ripening.
- **Castor oil**   Stimulation of the bowels to aid sympathetic contractions of the uterus was formerly used to try and induce labor. Women used to be prescribed oil baths and an enema which was, and still is, sometimes effective in starting contractions, although it will also leave you feeling exhausted and debilitated at the start of labor. If you want to try it, take a third of a glass mixed with orange juice. Be prepared for copious diarrhea.
- **Curry**   A purgative which works in the same way as castor oil.
- **Sweep of membranes**   Your midwife can help by giving you a vaginal examination and then sweeping her finger round inside your cervix so that the lower membranes become detached. It can only be done when your cervix is ripe. Studies have demonstrated that this can induce labor within three days in two-thirds of women (Allot 1993, Grant 1993).

- **Homeopathy** It is certainly worth trying Caulophyllum 30, available from homeopathic pharmacies only, every hour until contractions start, and continuing until labor is well established. If nothing happens after two days you can try taking Caulophyllum 200. Make it more powerful by adding a tablet to a glass of water, sipping it gradually until there is a third left and topping it up with water again. You can repeat the cycle ad infinitum so that the Caulophyllum becomes more and more diluted and, in homeopathic terms, stronger. It is best to avoid eating and drinking around the same time as taking the tablets. Although this does not work for everyone, for many women it provides a safe pleasant way to start labor, which is often quick and efficient. If medical induction becomes necessary, Caulophyllum can help to make it quicker. This treatment may take two or three days to work.
- **Acupuncture** Treatment from an acupuncturist does work, although again it may take several days. Ask for a retaining pin in your ear, (a bit like a seed taped in place) so that you can continue to apply pressure to stimulate contractions yourself. (See also pressure points on pages 110–111.)

• *Cathy Doberska* •

I wish I had known before my first birth that the process of induction can be very painful. Everyone I have spoken to since, who has had both induced and spontaneous labors, has said that the induced ones were far more painful. It made no difference whether the induced labor was the first or fourth delivery.

My induced contractions were unbelievably painful, with the start of labor feeling like being thrown into a brick wall at high speed. They were "square" shaped on the monitor strip rather than building up gradually and were very irregular. The Demerol was horrible, but at least I lost all sense of time passing . . .

It took a normal birth to restore my faith in the natural processes!

Chapter Four

PSYCHOLOGY OF LABOR

People who are familiar with the progress of birth may not recognize the potential of a woman to be in control during labor. They know how overwhelming a force it can be and are familiar with seeing people in labor who may appear to be (or actually are) out of control. However, control, or ability not to be panicked by the process, is vital to many women. Several studies have shown that it is not the level of pain which is most significant to women in labor, but the mastery of the situation. Labor is regarded with more satisfaction if a woman feels she remained in control – whatever that may mean for her – rather than if it was pain-free. Some women may feel they control it best by choosing to have full pain relief.

Several factors are recognized to increase psychological pain in labor. There are many more tactics that you can use to overcome it, although you may need determination. Those things that can affect psychological pain include:

- Disturbance
- Focusing on the labor
- Environment
- Fear
- Ignorance
- Caregivers
- Induction.

· *Disturbance* ·

Animals commonly seek out quiet, dark, peaceful places to give birth. Not even expensive racehorses are expected to give birth in an animal hospital. Interestingly, if horses are intended to foal somewhere other than on their home territory they have to be moved at least two or three weeks before the date they are due. If animals are disturbed during the course of labor, it can interrupt the process and even result in the babies being born dead.

Tests with mice showed that deliberate disturbance – handling them, moving them from their cage to a bowl smelling of cats, and moving them from bowl to bowl could make labor last one-and-a-half times as long as those in a control group that were left alone (Newton N 1966, Newton N 1968). Those who were moved from cage to bowl and back delivered twice as many babies in the cage as in the bowl, and one-and-a-half times as many mice pups were born dead, most of those in the bowl.

When monkeys in labor were deliberately stressed by having lights shone in their eyes, their toes clamped, or a white-coated researcher jump up and down in front of them, their blood pressures and heart rates rose and fetal hearts slowed.

Although no one is likely to clamp your toes, the effect of moving from home to the hospital, or from maternity ward to delivery room, or transferring to a strange environment that you are unlikely to know well (you will not even know which room you will be in), can undoubtedly increase stress levels and it is well known that labor may slow or stop on arrival, however intense it may have been on the way there.

Of course for some there is the relief of putting responsibility into someone else's hands. Laboring at home without anyone to reassure you that everything is proceeding well and normally can be stressful in itself. However, most delivery rooms will never look or feel like home, no matter how hard people have tried to make them comfortable. The balance of power shifts so that even those used to exercising power and control in their everyday lives can find it hard not to be overcome by a sense of being on someone else's territory. Although staff are all individuals and not "them," they are familiar with the surroundings and each other and can predict to a certain extent how they will behave or what will happen in a given situation. If you already know your midwife, a lot of stress will be removed already. She can act as your interpreter and go-between and help to make you feel comfortable in those surroundings. If not, you have to establish a trusting relationship rapidly.

Other aspects of the labor ward may be disconcerting; for example, you may hear other women in labor. Although they may find the noise helpful and it may not indicate great distress, it can be highly unnerving for you and your partner. In a community, it would be most unlikely to have two women in labor at the same time – and even more unlikely that they would be within earshot of each other. However, having laboring women together is the *raison d'être* of maternity units, and these noises as well as all the other unfamiliar noises cannot be underestimated as a cause of stress. Even the fact that you do not know when the sound of footsteps will end at your door, or what a knock on the door precedes, can be perturbing.

Preparation, rehearsal, and familiarity will decrease the anxieties to some extent and many women say that in advanced labor they were unaware of who was there and cared less. However, it is in the early part that women who are sensitive – and sensitivity is heightened in most people during labor – find establishing themselves in the hospital a trial. It is literally a testing time; on admission you are likely to have your temperature, blood pressure and urine tested. Most units will want to measure the baby's heart rate via a continuous electrical fetal heart monitor, and you will probably be given a vaginal examination. All these things can be quite daunting if done as routine at any time – during pregnancy for example.

• *Caregivers* •

One of the factors that is crucial to the way that you feel about your labor, and the degree to which you are able to relax, is that of the caregiver who is with you in labor. Again and again studies have highlighted the fact that she or he can make all the difference. A sympathetic, caring, positive midwife can help you through the pain of labor. An unsympathetic midwife whose behavior may be technically faultless can slow progress dramatically. Unfortunately, you may not be able to choose your midwife unless you employ an independent midwife, although the value of knowing your midwife before labor starts is being recognized increasingly by midwifery managers, and schemes being set up now promote the chances of this happening.

The majority of midwives are exceptionally nice people with whom it is a pleasure to share labor and from whom you will be sad to be parted. It must be said that there are some – either because they have a different philosophy from you, or due to problems in their personal lives, or simply because things are not going well for them that day – who will not make you feel at ease. They may make you feel fearful and imply that you are making a fuss or that the way you want to do things is unreasonable.

If you feel instinctively that you and the midwife with you in labor have different aims then you must ask for a change. Your partner can leave the room and ask to speak to whoever is in charge; explain the problem pleasantly and you will be allocated someone else. This can feel hard to do in an unfamiliar environment but it is important; remember that if you find that your caregiver is hindering rather than helping your labor it will last longer, feel more painful, you may need more medication and intervention, and it can distress your baby.

Another way around possible problems, which requires prior planning, is to have a birth supporter as well as your partner there – as discussed on pages 54–57. This can be highly effective in easing stress and pain in labor.

• *Helping to Minimize Labor Pain* •

There are a number of things that help to reduce the awareness of labor pain. Most are under your control, although some, such as the confidence engendered by having been through labor pain before, or previous experience of nongynecological pain, obviously are not. Many of the techniques are more useful if they have been learned and practiced in pregnancy, although it is quite possible to pick up a simple and effective breathing technique in labor, and one of the most effective ways of decreasing pain and increasing the efficiency of the labor is by remaining upright.

Here are some of the things that are helpful and that do not require prior organization.

Movement
- Remaining upright, moving around, and changing position frequently. Walking up and down stairs, if available, can be useful too.
- Other physical movements: swaying from hip to hip, rotating the hips, pacing up and down.
- Rubbing above or below the pain, stamping, gripping something hard or using one hand to grip tightly while relaxing the rest of your body (Although hardly a relaxation technique, biting hard on something, or digging nails into a partner's hand have been known to help.)

Breathing
- Breathing slowly, in through your nose and out through your mouth, concentrating on the out breath, can work remarkably well and is easy to remember. It can help to push your abdomen out on the outward breath.

Using Water

- Water – bathing or showering – can be soothing and relaxing, and is very useful for labor even if not planning a water birth. You should have access to a bath or shower in most units; a shower is useful if you want to remain upright.
- It can help to get someone else to direct a jet at the area which seems most painful, or you could try sitting back to front on a plastic chair, letting water flow down your back.

Eating and Drinking

It is valuable to eat and drink to provide energy for the intense work your body is doing (see pages 72–75). Do not worry about being sick; although unpleasant, it is normal and can help to move the baby down and relax perineal muscles in the second stage.

Distractions

Physical Distraction

- Concentrating on doing something else can be very useful. Do anything that appeals, such as going for a walk, visiting a garden center, or indulging in the nesting instinct by cleaning or getting things ready. It is best to conserve some energy for later but it can be satisfying to actually achieve something. Ironing is particularly useful as an ironing board is the right height to lean over during a contraction.
- You may find it helpful *not* to focus on the labor in the early stages and to carry on as normal, or construct things to do. Labor will seem shorter and less painful this way. There will come a point when you will have to pay attention to it, but try to delay it as long as you possibly can.

Mental Distraction

- You can distract yourself by concentrating on something else such as talking, watching a film or television programme, or listening to music. In the later stages, when contractions demand a lot of attention, you may like to try mental techniques often used by people in pain. Examples include counting backwards from a hundred in groups of three (vary the number); retracing a familiar route in your imagination; picturing people or places; visualising an action connected with your work; spelling out words as you hear them on the radio; imagining packing a suitcase, rearranging furniture, painting your house different colors; or making something up in your mind. You could use your surroundings; counting the tiles on the wall, tracing patterns on the wallpaper or tiles on the floor.

- Another way of using mental distraction is to concentrate hard on one thing. You could close your eyes and fill your mind with a color that you especially like, listen hard to music, or just stare hard at a flower, picture, or any one thing in the room. A candle flame can be a good thing to focus on.

- You can also use words to help you, either mentally or aloud. Women often find that repetition is valuable; they may recite prayers, or nursery rhymes, sing songs or chant, or recite poetry over and over again. Words can include oaths, psalms, or complete phrases such as: "I can do it; it is going to be fine."

- You can also rise above it; try to disengage yourself from your body and look down on it from above, or try and imagine that the areas that are painful do not belong to you.

- Alternatively, you can employ the opposite technique to distraction and concentrate fully on contractions, welcoming each one as it nears the birth, and thinking hard about the sensation rather than the pain they cause. Try to analyze what is happening within your body; see if you can visualize your baby and what is happening to it inside you. See if you can feel your cervix opening; visualize it doing so and imagine it opening up still further.

- Remind yourself that it is normal to feel pain with contractions and then for it to cease in between (continuous pain may indicate that something is wrong). Remember that it will not last forever and may all be over by tomorrow.

- Buy time by dealing with each contraction at a time. Do not anticipate by thinking that you will not be able to cope if it gets worse, or that you cannot stand much more of this. Look forward to and make the most of the break between contractions. If pain relief is suggested (rather than you asking for it) delay it for a few contractions at a time – say, five more. Do not accept it to make anyone else feel better, or be led to believe that you had better have it now because it may not be available later.

Making a Noise

- Making a noise in labor can be instinctive but may also be governed by cultural norms. In China or among the Bedouins making a noise in labor is considered disgraceful and likely to bring shame on the family and women are expected to conduct their labor in silence. In other cultures, it is considered important to scream, shout, and make as much noise as possible.

- Experienced midwives are able to tell how a woman's labor is progressing without examining her, partly by her appearance and the way she is behaving, but also by listening to the sounds she makes. Some of the sounds recognized (McKay 1990) include sighing, moaning, and groaning, which are coping sounds, considered self-comforting and soothing.

  The noise typical of the second stage is guttural, a grunt with an "uhh" sound, and can sound primal or animalistic. You may recognize this stage yourself if you hear yourself start to grunt as you breath out. This sound is quite involuntary and is caused by a catch in the throat. It signals the start of the expulsive stage, although you may not feel the urge to push yet.

- You may make other noises – whining like a puppy or crying like a baby – which signal pain and distress and tell your care-givers that you are scared, or afraid of losing control.

- Outright shrieking, yelling, and screaming probably does indicate loss of control, unless you feel that this is normal in your society. Midwives should move quickly to help you.

- The question of environment and the issue of making a noise in labor arise here. Some women are glad to give birth at home because they feel they can be as uninhibited as they like and make whatever noise will help. Others find the idea of making a noise that neighbors might hear inhibiting.

- The noises women make in labor can be quite disturbing to others – particularly partners. It can be quite hard for fathers to understand that a woman making a noise in labor is not necessarily in great distress and that she finds it both instinctive and helpful. Midwives too can find it alarming and offer pain relief as a way not only to help what may seem (but not be) agony, but also to silence the woman.

Partner Suggestions

Suggestions as to how your partner can help you are on pages 57–61. His presence can be invaluable even if he says or does little.

Chapter Five

ENVIRONMENT

The place where you give birth and the people you have attending you can make a lot of difference to the way in which you experience labor and the amount of pain you feel.

• *Environment and Pain in Labor* •

There are two pieces of interesting evidence relating to pain in labor.

The first study refers directly to home birth, and deals with pain levels felt by 282 women giving birth at home in Canada, compared with those of women giving birth in hospital. They asked both the mothers and the fathers to rate pain levels. The hospital group rated childbirth pain significantly higher than the home-birth group. In the home-birth group, women considered the pain to be less than the males and in the hospital birth group the females rated pain higher than the males. The study was not able to conclude whether the home-birth women actually felt less pain or were simply more tolerant, but it is interesting that the men rated pain as being greater when they had more responsibility for helping at the birth.

The second study, in Denmark, monitored the levels of pain relief between women giving birth in a consultant unit and those giving birth in an alternative birth center (ABC; which would translate roughly to a midwifery-led unit). The ABC was physically linked to the obstetrics unit. This study is of particular interest because it includes women who had chosen the ABC but had to deliver in the obstetrics unit because the ABC was full at the time. Much less pain relief was used in the ABC.

Twenty-four women who had chosen the ABC, but who had to give birth in the obstetrics unit, required Demerol in the same measure as the women who had chosen the obstetrics unit. This suggests that place of delivery, together with its attendant philosophy, policies, and way of practicing can overwhelm women's ability to cope.

The authors concluded that the ABC was able to protect first-time mothers and young women, so they gained belief in their ability to cope and give birth without pain relief, except in the second stage.

• *Hospital or Home?* •

Comparatively little work has been published on this, perhaps because it would be invidious to show that different midwives helped mothers to different outcomes, and certainly because in the headlong rush to get women to deliver in the hospital the soft data ("how she feels about it") and quite a lot of the hard (cesarean-section rate, etc.) have been wilfully ignored. Although the tide regarding the issue of home birth has begun to turn, it is still not generally recognized that statistically, the infant death rate in a hospital setting is greater than in planned, attended home births.

A survey of statistics by Rona Campbell and Alison MacFarlane of the National Perinatal Epidemiology Unit 1987 found, among other things, that:

- The statistical association between the increase in the proportion of hospital deliveries and the fall in crude perinatal mortality rate seems unlikely to be explained by a cause and effect relation.
- There is no evidence to support the claim that the safest policy is for all women to deliver in the hospital.
- There is some evidence, although not conclusive, that morbidity (disease or abnormality) is higher among mothers and babies cared for in an institutional setting. For some women the iatrogenic risk (that caused by the process of diagnosis or treatment) associated with institutional delivery may be greater than any benefit conferred, but this has yet to be proven.
- A majority of women who have experienced both home and hospital deliveries prefer to have their babies at home, although this may include a disproportionate number of women who have sought home delivery after a hospital delivery with which they were dissatisfied.

This data is mostly concerned with the crude measurable outcome of mortality and morbidity in babies and their mothers, and largely does not reflect how women feel about the experience of hospital as opposed to home birth.

If you have always believed that hospital birth is necessarily safer, it can be quite a shock to realize that the reverse may be true. More information is available in my book, *Home Birth*.

· *Choosing Home Birth* ·

Women choose home birth for the following reasons:

- They feel more relaxed in the privacy of their own home and labor is less stressful
- They feel free to do whatever they want and are not inhibited by the hospital setting, which is alien to them
- They have had previous bad experiences with hospital deliveries
- They cannot have continuous electronic fetal monitoring
- They are more likely to know their midwife
- They can eat and drink freely
- Time limits on stages of labor are much less likely to be enforced; there is no way of attaching a drip to artificially stimulate contractions; and Pitocin cannot be used
- There is plenty for fathers to do and couples will not be parted after the birth
- Children can be present if wished and it is less disruptive to their lives
- You can have whoever you want with you at the birth
- The baby is less disturbed if it is born into its home and both the mother and baby are at much lower risk of infection that can be acquired in the hospital
- They receive individual attention from midwives during pregnancy and at the birth; the midwife will not be caring for other women in labor at the same time.

· *Marie Coveney* ·

With my first birth I accepted the status quo and had shared care with my GP and the hospital, and I accepted that I would not know the midwife who was to help me deliver. Afterward, I heard of other people who had used independent midwives and I really hankered after the continuity of care that they seemed to have had and wished that I could justify the cost.

When I was pregnant with my second child I wanted to plan a home birth, and a community midwife came to see me to talk about it. Although she is pro home birth, she advised me against it when she learned that I had lost 1500 ml of blood after Elizabeth's birth and had needed a blood transfusion, because she felt that it might happen again. I was quite bothered by this and spoke to a lot of experienced midwives who all said that it was unlikely unless I was surrounded by people who were expecting it to happen. I was afraid that if I went ahead with the home-birth plan, they would find a spurious reason to take me in due to their anxiety, and there was obviously no way that I would be allowed a physiological third stage.

We talked to quite a few independent midwives and then met Melanie who I knew had been a prenatal teacher before becoming a midwife, and who was strongly in favor of informed choice. I knew that I would feel safer at home with her than going to the hospital. I really liked her, and so we scheduled with her.

It was so nice to see just her and one other midwife for prenatal visits, all of which were at home. She used to come and check me on our sofa; her visits never lasted less than an hour and a half so that I was able to discuss everything that concerned me; and she could explain exactly what she was doing. I never had to see my obstetrician; it was so different from having just ten minutes with a different person each time. Melanie was very supportive of the various preparations that I made for the birth. I planned a water birth, also used self-hypnosis as preparation for the birth, and reflexology, which helped my insomnia. I also took homeopathic remedies for my hemoglobin levels; all of these steps helped me to feel in control.

In the end it was very quick. Elizabeth was spending the weekend with my mother. I was just two days overdue, the house was very quiet, and I felt ready when I was awakened a couple of times by crampy period-type pains in the night. I went back to sleep each time but in the morning I got very mild early contractions every 5 minutes, lasting 15 seconds. Then, when I was having breakfast I found that I had to stand up and sway my pelvis from side to side.

I went up to tell Paul that this was it, and we started to put our plans into action. I intended to have a bath, call Melanie, put the TENS on and then fill the pool. While I was in the bath I had two intense contractions and so we called her right away. She said she would be there in half an hour and that was it; my body was pushing although I was trying not to. For the next half hour I was on the bed in the knee-chest position with my bottom in the air, trying to stop the baby arriving before the midwife. We didn't have time for the TENS or the pool, let alone the Arnica or the Rescue Remedy. I told Paul just to get a plastic sheet. He was very agitated, saying "you can't be pushing, that's the second stage!"

There was only a short break between contractions and as soon as Melanie arrived she put on her gloves and then helped me to have the baby instead of holding it back. She managed to get me upright and Alice was born into dim lighting in the quiet presence of just three people, half an hour later. I was in a supported standing-squat (supported by my poor husband) when Melanie passed her up to me: my baby born by my own efforts, nobody got her out for me. It was blissful.

There was a moment after that when I seemed to be bleeding quite a lot and Melanie asked Paul to get the Pitocin out of the fridge. Melanie was so calm and by the time he came back with it, the bleeding had stopped and I didn't need it, so we were able to breathe a sigh of relief.

There was no hurry to get us cleaned up or for Alice to have all her checks and tests; nobody was working to any agenda but our own and we didn't have to be hurried off to the postnatal ward. The placenta followed after about twenty minutes and then we had a cup of tea and a chocolate biscuit.

I had a small second degree tear that we all agreed could be left unstitched. It was uncomfortable for only about two days and I am sure that my recovery was helped by Arnica 200.

Alice and I had a nice warm bath together, got into our own bed, and she had a blissful long sleep. We had postpartum care over the next twenty-eight days

For us, paying to get the chance of a better birth experience was worth every penny.

• *Home Birth* •

Many more women would like to have their babies at home than actually do. The reasons they are deterred include pressure from family and friends, talk of risk of complication or outright denial by obstetricians, discouragement from midwifery staff who may be very apprehensive if they have no experience of home birth, and lack of a mothers' network – they may not know anyone of their age who has given birth at home.

In the United States, home birth is rare, and you will need to take the initiative if you want to arrange one. Doctors usually will not attend a home birth, so you will probably need to find a midwife. To find a midwife in your area, contact the Midwives Alliance of North America for further information (see resources, page 149).

Studies have shown that planned home births attended by experienced midwives are safe, and midwives are skilled in identifying and dealing with minor complications. Midwives screen women during prenatal care and refer those with serious health problems to an obstetrician.

The best place for you to have your baby is where you will feel most comfortable, whether that is in a high-tech hospital unit or at home. It is important to fully explore the options open to you locally before making a decision, and to know that you can change your mind at any point until you have had the baby. The woman's feelings are of prime importance. She is the one giving birth and only she will know what feels best to her.

Many women have stated that they would like to have their babies at home, but their partners are opposed to it. This can be related to male anxiety about having to cope alone and an often-expressed alarm about mess. Men are not as used as women to dealing with blood loss and can find it distressing. However, they do not have to give birth or even be present when birth takes place. It seems more important for a woman to give birth at home if that is where she feels happiest, than to subject her to the distress she may feel at having to go to a hospital.

• *Karen Long* •

I had my first child, Ffion, in the hospital, and ended up with forceps, which I didn't enjoy. Almost worse, though, was the belt monitor, which I hated because it meant that I was restricted to lying on the bed. I felt all the control had been taken out of my hands the moment that it was put on.

I had my second, Joshua, in a Swiss hospital, which was a good experience. I had wanted to have him at home but we were concerned that we might not get an English-speaking midwife. In fact, the hospital staff proved to be very laid back and not too bothered about the monitoring. His birth was very quick, I had him in a pool in just two hours, even though he was 9½ pounds.

By the time I was expecting our next baby we were back in England and I wanted to have the baby at home, but Rob, my husband, said he wasn't happy about it. Untypically, I accepted that, but as pregnancy progressed I got more and more concerned about actually getting to the hospital because it looked as though the birth might be very quick and it takes Rob forty-five minutes to get back from work. I worried about who would take me if he couldn't and what I would do with the children.

I went to the hospital to talk to a senior midwife about having a water birth, which they were happy to do, but it was agreed to with restrictions, including monitoring. She asked if I had considered having the baby at home and I also spoke to an prenatal teacher about it. Then I spoke to Rob, explaining exactly what I was concerned about. He hadn't really realized but after he had thought about it, and a community midwife had explained the pros and cons, he was quite happy about it. She put all his fears to rest and explained that it was far more relaxing and that mess need not be a problem.

Once the plan was changed, which was not difficult, I felt very happy and found that I was looking forward to the birth with excitement instead of dreading it. I spoke to a couple of friends who had had babies at home and got some ideas from them and felt much more content.

When the day came, I woke at 4:30 in the morning with very mild contractions every ten minutes. By 6:30 they were still not painful and coming every seven minutes, but I called the midwives because I wanted them to know that it had started because I thought that it would be very quick.

In fact, due to changing shifts, four midwives arrived which was nice because I had lots of attention, although I was indignant to hear them discussing who would be on duty tomorrow since I felt sure that I was going to have my baby that day. They all left and one, Marina, said that she was just going to collect some equipment and would be back within an hour. She suggested that I have some breakfast and a bath in the meantime. She examined me before she went and found I was 3 cm dilated, which I had been for a week, and that the head was high which was a surprise; I had been told it was low.

The examination may have stirred things up because shortly after she left I had a sudden, very definite contraction. I canceled the breakfast and got in the bath immediately. I had a friend with me and she stayed with me in the bathroom while Rob got the bedroom ready. By then, the contractions were coming every two minutes and I asked Rob to ask Marina to come back right away. I found the bath very relaxing and then got out to put my TENS machine on. Marina arrived with nitrous oxide and oxygen at 9:45 and I used it immediately, sitting upright at the head of the bed. This helped to bring the head down very quickly and then Marina suggested I try being on all fours on the bed, which felt really good. I sat upright for each contraction with Rob on one side of me and my friend on the other.

Contractions were coming thick and fast and I was finding it very hard and talking about Demerol when Marina asked if it would be all right to rupture the membranes. I could feel that they were causing a lot of pressure, so agreed. There was meconium in the waters and she said it would be best if the baby could be born as quickly as possible. I could hardly work out what was going on and asked if I could push. It only took four or five pushes after that and by 10:33 he was out, all 9 pounds 6 ounces and 21½ inches of him. It was very quick at the end, and the placenta followed almost immediately.

I did tear, so had some stitches, and then Ewan and I had a bath together which was wonderful. We then went back to our freshly made bed while my friend made tea downstairs. The children, who had gone to my friend's next door, had lunch and then came back to meet their new brother in their own home. I couldn't believe how lovely it was; it was absolutely magical and very special.

Rob was surprised by how pleased he was that we had him at home. He found that he was more able to be in control and take a more active part, helping the midwife and being on his own territory.

This is our last birth and the best. We would definitely recommend home birth.

Chapter Six

PREPARING FOR LABOR

• *Birth Partner and/or Supporter* •

Although it is not generally realized, one of the things that can make the biggest difference to the way labor goes is who you choose to have with you. You may think that this is obviously the baby's father, and certainly the general expectation nowadays is that the father will, or even should, be present at the birth of his baby. However, it may not be as simple as that and there can be various reasons for inviting someone else as well, or instead.

For some women, the baby's father is not available to be a birth partner and they will be encouraged to have someone else with them. It is perfectly possible to give birth attended only by midwifery or medical staff, and you may develop a close relationship with them. Some women prefer to not have anyone else involved and they should be free to do this, although it may be even more valuable to have met and come to trust a midwife beforehand.

The current expectation that the father should be present at the birth is a change in custom which is comparatively recent, and goes contrary to the way birth has been conducted for thousands of years among the vast majority of cultures. One of the reasons we have so little information about birth practices historically is because men were never allowed to be present, and customs were not written (men being more likely to be literate). In the past, when the majority of births took place at home, the father would be nearby, but not often in the birth room, except by accident at the moment of birth.

Nowadays, when the position has been reversed, many men are delighted to be there when their children are born, and describe the moment in touching terms as being the highlight of their lives. But even those men for whom it ultimately came to mean so much may have been reluctant to be there beforehand, and others, perhaps feeling the instinct that led to thousands of years of tradition, definitely did not wish to be present. This can create a real dilemma. Should a man trust his better judgment and deprive his wife or partner of the support that she badly wants and deserves, or should he conform to society's expectation and be with her throughout labor, despite deep feelings of unease? The problem is exacerbated by the fact that many very reluctant fathers, when compelled to be birth supporters, found that they wouldn't have missed it for anything.

It is not only the man who may feel strongly that birth is women's business. A mother may feel it too and prefer not to have him with her at the birth. She may also find, during the course of labor, that although she opted for his companionship, his presence becomes irritating or inhibiting in the event and she would like him to leave. It would be hard to deny a man the opportunity to see his child born, but as Tricia Anderson observes, "a person's physical presence does not always mean that they are giving support" (Anderson 1996), and although there are no hard and fast rules, it seems that the mother – without whom the child cannot be born – should have the ultimate choice.

If a couple are not in mutual agreement it will be hard to come to a conclusion as to who should be present at the birth. You may want other people as well or instead of your partner – perhaps your mother, sister, or friend. In many units there is no limit as to who can attend, although it should be remembered that the more there are the slower labor may be, and you may not feel like fulfilling the role of performance artist when it comes to it.

In this situation, you may find that you are not being supported sufficiently and have little opportunity for the privacy which can be essential in allowing birth to take place naturally. If you want a lot of family or friends with you, it is important to agree with them beforehand that they will leave the room if you ask.

Some units discourage the presence of more than one birth partner. If you would like more, it will help to negotiate in advance.

One solution can be to have an experienced woman birth supporter with you who is not necessarily related. Compelling evidence in a number of studies shows that the continued support of such a person can:
- reduce the need for pain relief, including epidurals
- result in fewer forceps or vacuum extraction deliveries
- result in fewer babies born by cesarean section
- result in babies born in better condition.

There did not appear to be any disadvantages in terms of labor, birth, or the babies, but there were other benefits such as:
- women found the experience of birth more positive

- women felt less tense during labor
- there was less damage to the perineum
- more women breastfed their babies for six weeks or more
- fewer women were found to have postpartum depression when assessed when the baby was six weeks old
- women had less difficulty in mothering
- the relationship between the father and the midwife was better.

Nowadays, although one can be reasonably sure of having one or more midwives present at the birth, pressure on time and the needs of other laboring women may mean that they cannot be with you throughout labor. It is, however, possible that you may be able to ask your own experienced birth supporter to be with you, who will help you throughout labor and bring the advantages mentioned.

If this is your first baby and you have no direct experience of labor, it can be hard to imagine how helpful the presence of a supporter can be. You may visualize labor as being a quiet, intimate affair where the presence of a relative stranger would be intrusive. Of course that may be true, but in reality having a birth supporter with you can be encouraging and reassuring. She will be a constant physical presence and be able to give advice and explanation and reassure you that things you did not expect are normal. This is particularly valuable during a new experience.

A woman who has had children can be more intuitive about how you are feeling and is able to offer physical support such as massage, drinks, and compresses. An extra pair of hands means that your partner can have a break to eat or drink or go to the bathroom. She will be able to make suggestions such as changing position, emptying your bladder, or having a bath, and is able to be more objective than perhaps family or friends. Her own experience will mean that she will be able to help you choose a specific course of action, seeing its advantages and disadvantages.

She will also be able to interpret your wishes to staff. Fathers, whose presence is often so welcome, cannot always be aware of the consequences of various obstetric procedures, despite prenatal education, and they find it more difficult to take the long view. The fact that obstetric interventions are reduced where women have birth supporters present suggests that medical staff are more likely to think twice – perhaps a birth supporter's presence means that they are happier to allow labor to take its course. Perhaps the reduction in anxiety levels means they are not needed, or the baby recognizes that its mother feels reassured. At any rate, the studies found that the supporter who supports both partners finds the father to be more supportive himself.

The idea of professional lay support is well established in the U.S. If you do not know anyone who could help you in this way you could try a prenatal teacher/birth educator – all of whom have a great interest in birth and would be delighted to be asked.

• *Suggestions for Birth Partners* •

If you are to be a birth partner it is important to discuss the birth in detail, see how the mother feels on all sorts of issues and hypothesize about possible events, such as what if it lasted longer than expected, would she prefer a cut to an episiotomy, would she like an epidural or prefer to be encouraged to manage without. Birth plans are valuable as evidence of what the mother would prefer, but are no substitute for discussion.

Beforehand
If the birth is planned for the hospital, try to visit beforehand. Look around and envisage what you will need to make yourselves comfortable there. Preplanning is not so crucial if you are having your baby at home, but there will be far more for you to do there, and it will be better to get ready as much as possible beforehand.
- Have plenty of food and drink ready. It is helpful for a woman to eat and drink during labor, and you will value it especially if labor is long and tiring. The hospital cafeteria may not be open, or your partner may not want you to leave.
- Take things for your own comfort: washing/shaving things, toothbrush, change of underwear; anything that might help when up all day and night engaged in hard physical exercise.
- Remember to have change ready for the pay phone. Cell phones are often not allowed in hospitals because they can interfere with signals from the monitors.
- If you have children, make sure there is someone to look after them, especially if they are to be present at the birth.
- Keep the car gas tank full.

The Birth
Your job is to support your partner positively and wholeheartedly because she will probably feel very vulnerable and will be dependent on you to help her get through the birth.

You will need to be her voice, to help her manage to do things the way that she wants, and to negotiate for her if necessary.

Going into the hospital with someone in labor (and to a lesser extent being with them in labor at home) can be daunting, especially if you are not familiar with the place or the people and have never even seen anyone in labor before. It is easy to become intimidated, to feel that the hospital staff have all the experience and so they know best. Being in a room with your partner, not knowing who is going to come in next or what they are going to say can be alarming. Even experienced birth supporters can find it daunting, not because they lack faith in a woman's ability to cope, or doubt that her body can do it, but because it is venturing somewhat into the unknown when the establishment seems to hold all the cards. Ideally, you and your partner will already know the midwife you are allocated, so that you will already have established a relationship of trust, be pleased to see each other, and feel confident that she already knows what your partner wants.

If the midwife is new to you, you will have to build up a relationship rapidly. It is important to do this, in order to make your partner feel confident that you are all working together as a team for her good and to create a positive atmosphere. The majority of midwives are exceptionally pleasant people, well used to making people feel at ease. However, it is well recognized that a minority are not necessarily so supportive, and may for various reasons not be encouraging, take a pessimistic view, withhold information, imply that the woman is making a fuss about nothing, exclude partners or not respond to questions, or deny women's feelings (Kirkham, Hunt).

If the midwife is feeling jaded you may need to support her, making her realize she is appreciated and that you want as much information and encouragement as possible. If, however, you feel it is unlikely that you will ever hit it off, then it is important to find a midwife with whom you feel comfortable. This can seem hard, but you will only have this labor once. It is not worth putting up with second best when it is only chance that has put you and the midwife together.

Going into the Hospital

Being at home with a woman in labor can create anxiety, particularly if you have no experience of women in labor. First-time parents are inclined to go into the hospital earlier than they need because they find it hard to recognize how advanced labor is, or be able to estimate how much longer it may take. Ideally, you will be able to call a midwife to come and see you and make that assessment for you. If not, concern about leaving too late, and the thought of having to deliver the baby yourself can make men panic and urge them to lose no time in reaching hospital.

Guidelines about when to go in are contained on pages 10–11. It is important, though, to be guided by her feelings rather than yours; to consider that you will not be as physically comfortable or free to do what you want in a hospital environment; that labor is likely to last several hours more; and to go in with a view to having the progress of labor checked with the possibility of going home, rather than letting everyone know that this is it, and then feeling obliged to stay there to save face.

Have faith in your ability to cope and continue to support and encourage her – and make sure you have the midwife's or doctor's number handy just in case the baby starts arriving rapidly.

How to Help
- Support and continual encouragement are vital; tell her how well she is doing, how brave she is being, that you will soon have your baby.
- Make sure that she continues to eat and drink; put things ready for her.
- Encourage her to alter position, and stay mainly upright. It is easy to get stuck in one position or avoid moving about if it strengthens contractions and increases pain, but labor will be over more quickly that way. You may need to remind her of this.
- It is important that she empties her bladder at least every hour; otherwise it can impede the progress of the baby down the birth canal. Remind her and help if she finds it difficult, particularly if she is asked to use a bedpan or there are other people in the room. She may feel less inhibited if they leave and you run the taps. It may be easier to do it in a shower.
- She may not want you to leave at all. Make sure there is someone with her if you have to go out for any reason, and return as quickly as possible.
- She may want you to leave, although this is unlikely if you are providing sensitive support. She may also become angry or swear at you and others. Try not to take it personally and do

not retaliate. If you are asked to leave, let her and the midwife know that you will be close by.

- Be prepared to do massage for long periods of time. (See pages 70–72.) This can be uncomfortable for you, and you may not be able to do it in the best position for your back. Minimize the strain as far as possible and be prepared for aching muscles later on.

- Do not consider that crossing the threshold of a maternity unit means you can only come out with a baby. It is much easier these days to go in for an assessment and then go back home if labor is going slowly, or if membranes have ruptured but the baby is fine. Go for a walk around the hospital if you don't want to leave entirely. It will help to get things in perspective, and walking helps labor to progress.

Making Decisions

Labor can throw up occasions where decisions have to be made, ranging from whether to go and have a cup of tea to the question of the need for a cesarean section. Even everyday choices can seem magnified in their intensity because of the nature of the situation and the loss of usual reference points. Clearly, the ultimate choice must rest with the mother, but you may need to be her interpreter and negotiator, particularly if she is too preoccupied to deal with it herself. Labor pain can demand such reserves of energy that there is little left over for rational thought or discussions.

You should be aware of what she feels on particular issues and should be able to speak for her. It is essential that you present her case to the staff and not the other way round. It is all too easy to become institutionalized and want to cooperate with hospital staff, running the risk of responding to them should they say "Just tell your wife we are going to do this, Mr. X". It is possible to be overawed by their knowledge (and for them to intend you to be) so that you comply with their wishes instead of those of your partner. You *must* remain on her side at all times.

Admittedly, it can be difficult to decide what to do if circumstances have compelled her to change her mind about something she has decided previously. For example, if she has been adamant about not having an epidural and now is insisting that she wants one, are you to agree or remind her of her wishes? In this case you might ask for a check of the dilation of cervix, remind her of her wishes, try every other form of pain relief, including bath or shower and ambulation. If she is still insistent ask three times in

Inner Traditions International, Ltd.
P.O. Box 388
Rochester, VT 05767
U.S.A.

If you wish to receive a copy of the latest INNER TRADITIONS INTERNATIONAL catalog and to be placed on our mailing list, please send us this card. It is important to print your name and address clearly.

Name _____ Phone _____

Address _____

City _____ State _____ Zip _____

Country _____ Email address _____

Order at 1-800-246-8648 • Fax (802) 767-3726
E-mail: orders@InnerTraditions.com • Web site: www.InnerTraditions.com

total – and then agree. Point out it will take twenty to thirty minutes to set up – and see how she feels when the anaesthetist arrives. By then labor may only last a bit longer – and you don't have to have the epidural just because you have requested it some time ago.

It can be very hard to see someone you love in pain, and so you may want her to have pain relief to ease your anxiety as well as her own. However, she may want support rather than drugs: don't press them on her; she will let you know if she can't manage without.

Other decisions can be hard to make, too, especially if you feel you lack the knowledge on which to base them. It can help to consider the following points so that you and your partner can make the best decision in the circumstances. To make them easy to remember, learn them as an acronym, BRAN:

- What are the <u>B</u>enefits?
- What are the <u>R</u>isks?
- What are the <u>A</u>lternatives?
- What will happen if we do <u>N</u>othing?

It is always important to trust her instinct. Do not be pressured into agreeing to something that either of you have reservations about, thinking that you will worry about the consequences later. There is almost always time to consider. If the situation is a real emergency you will be in no doubt and there will be little time for debate.

Do consider the long-term consequences. Although at the time, getting the baby out can seem to be of paramount importance, the memories will last a lifetime and it is important that a woman should be able to look back at the birth with pride knowing that she was in control and that she dictated the way it went, given the circumstances.

· *The Position of the Baby* ·

It is often suspected that a largely sedentary lifestyle, interspersed with periods of exercise, are fitting us less well for giving birth than the more active lifestyles of women who lived before the invention of washing machines, dishwashers, and carpeting.

Up until fairly recently, life was physically hard for the majority of women, who even if they weren't working outside the home, would spend a lot of time and energy on their feet, or scrubbing floors. Only wealthy women – famously too refined to be good at giving birth – had leisure to spend their lives sitting over embroidery or needlework.

Peasant women, who customarily worked up until the very last moment, had a reputation for giving birth with ease, and although they often gave birth in hugely unsanitary conditions they often seemed to fare better. Although there were many tragic exceptions, there are stories of women going off to the fields with just a pair of scissors and a reel of thread as the essential equipment for delivery, which shows an anticipation of birth being simple as well as an enviable degree of self-reliance. Gélis relates the story of a French woman at the beginning of the twentieth century who went to work in the fields equipped in this way and returned with a new baby perched in her wheelbarrow on top of the beets. Apparently all her children were born that way.

Although it would be simplistic to suggest that all women should take up hoeing or floor scrubbing as a way of life in pregnancy, it can be a good idea to think about the position that the baby is in during late pregnancy because some positions are more favorable than others – leading to a quicker, easier, straightforward labor.

It used to be the case that midwives and obstetricians were not too concerned about the position in which a baby was lying provided it was head down, because experience showed that it would probably rotate into a favorable position during labor. Recently, though, the work of Jean Sutton and Valerie El Halta has been examined with interest because they suggest ways in which mothers can help to turn their babies into the best position before labor begins. This much reduces the chances of long, painful, inefficient labors with severe backache, such as when the back of the baby's head is against its mother's spine (occipito-posterior or OP) or other malpositions, some of which require cesarean section.

Ideal Position of Baby for Labor

The ideal position for a baby to be in as labor starts is left occipito-anterior (LOA), when the back of the baby's head is against its mother's hip, so that its curved back can be felt along the left-hand side of the abdomen between the hips and mother's navel. In this position it is able to turn its head through 45 degrees towards its mother's front. The head can slip through the left side under her sacrum, with the baby's chin on its chest and its shoulders crossing the pelvis from the mother's back to front.

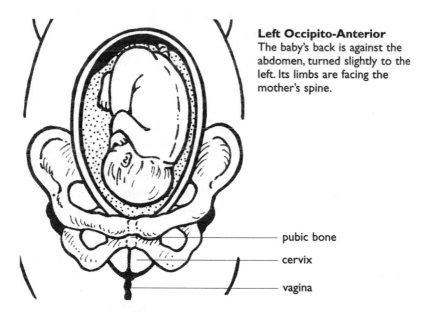

Left Occipito-Anterior
The baby's back is against the abdomen, turned slightly to the left. Its limbs are facing the mother's spine.

pubic bone

cervix

vagina

Late pregnancy contractions help to move the baby's head further into the pelvis so that when it is fully engaged only one-fifth can be felt above the pelvic brim. This may be felt as painful contractions: "entering pains". The leading part of the head – known as the vertex – is now near the level of the ischial spines. Once it is past the brim and into the cavity of the pelvis, the baby's head turns so that the back of its head is against the mother's pubic bone (symphysis pubis). As the baby moves further down, the back of the head is pushed below the symphysis pubis and backward, so that when the baby is born its face is facing its mother's anus. The baby's shoulders, which are now in the pelvic cavity, are across the pelvis from back to front so that one shoulder lies under the pubic bone. At the moment of birth the baby's neck is twisted because its head is in a line with the other shoulder that is under the sacrum. As the head becomes free, the baby turns it so that it now faces its mother's thigh. The shoulder under the pubic arch is born first and then the other shoulder slips from under the sacrum. After this, the body is easily born.

It is much easier to visualize the passage of the baby through the pelvis if you have the opportunity to play with a doll and model of a pelvis, available at most prenatal classes. Ask to experiment with them, as it can make the whole process much clearer.

However, not all babies adopt an LOA position before birth. Roughly 3 percent are not even head down. Pelvises are different shapes. Some are wider at the brim but narrow in the outlet, others are narrow at the brim, some have different angles at the sacrum, the sacrum can be more or less curved, and there are many other variants which can affect the process of birth. Even so, the ability of the baby's skull bones to move over one another and the give of the mother's ligaments in labor can add or subtract several centimeters to the diameters and make theoretically difficult dimensions perfectly possible.

At the start of labor, roughly 75 percent of babies are in the LOA position and its symmetrical opposite ROA (when the baby's back is on its mother's right side). These positions bode well.

OP Positions

Occipito-posterior positions – when the baby's back is against the mother's back, either directly (spine to spine OP) or to the left or right of the spine (LOP) or (ROP) – are less favorable. This is because it is harder for the head to enter the pelvis and it will have

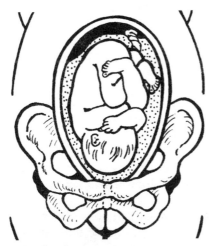

Right Occipito-Posterior
The baby's back is against the mother's spine with its limbs at the front of the abdomen. Its back is turned slightly to the right.

to rotate through 135 degrees instead of 45 degrees when it is in the pelvic cavity in order to be born with its face facing the anus. If the baby is unable to turn it may be born with the face to the pubis (persistent occipito-posterior: POP), but there is increased likelihood of it becoming stuck with its head partially rotated, which reduces the chances of vaginal birth.

OP labors are notorious for the backache that they can cause. Although this can be helped with TENS, they are likely to be longer and much more painful than an OA labor. This is because the head does not fit well to the cervix so that oxytocin production is not constant and so can produce short, painful but irregular contractions. Labor can seem to last for ages with little progress apparently being made.

Altering the Baby's Position

Fortunately, there are ways of helping a baby turn from an OP position to OA before labor starts – providing you know what position the baby is in. Always ask your midwife which position she thinks the baby is in, although you can tell for yourself if you are one of the 15 to 30 percent of women whose babies are OP. If it is a first baby you should start trying to get it to shift position at around 34 weeks which is when the position starts to become fixed. Women who have already had one or more children can leave it until 37 weeks as their uterine muscles are likely to be looser giving the baby more room to move.

Signs of an OP baby include:

- The baby kicks at the front
- There is a saucer-shaped dip around your navel
- The head does not engage; usual is at about 36 weeks with a first baby; later with subsequent ones
- Pressure on your bladder may mean you have to urinate frequently. You may feel as if you have a urinary tract infection because there may also be a constant pressure on the symphisis pubis and a low backache.
- Your midwife may find it hard to hear the baby's heartbeat.

The steps that you can take to persuade the baby to turn include:

- Rocking your pelvis backwards and forwards several times a day. Try this standing and in the all-fours position.
- Spend twenty minutes, three times a day, with your knees on the ground, your bottom in the air and your head resting on your folded arms (the knee-chest position).
- Try lying backwards over a big board at a 45-degree angle so that your knees are in the air and your head is on a cushion at ground level. This should be done several times a day for thirty minutes at a time, if possible.
- Try having warm baths and gently encouraging the baby to roll over. Talking to it, telling it why you want it to turn, and visualizing it in the right position have been found to help greatly, according to Valerie El Halta.
- Valerie El Halta also finds that adopting the knee-chest position for forty-five minutes in early labor can help to turn babies who are in an OP position.
- Jean Sutton recommends making sure that a woman's knees are always lower than her hips in late pregnancy. She has observed that modern seating – which forces the pelvis to tip backward

rather than forward, as with standing or forward positions – prevents the baby from entering the pelvic brim in an OA position. She suggests sitting upright on hard chairs with backs, or putting a firm cushion underneath the bottom and lower back if sitting on a sofa, to make yourself more upright.

You can also lie forward over beanbags to watch television or use one of the backless chairs with a tilted seat and lower pad on which to rest the knees.

- Swimming on your front, yoga classes, and a Pregnancy Rocker (a rocking stool designed to help improve the baby's position) can all help, as well as treatment with acupuncture or homeopathy.

None of these methods are guaranteed to turn an OP baby, but there is evidence to show that they have worked for some people. They are well worth trying because success could make a big difference to your labor.

• *Birth Plans* •

Birth plans – originally scoffed at – are now a recognized part of the interaction between a mother and the maternity services. A recent survey suggested that as many as of 70 percent of women used them to prepare for labor and to clarify their views on the way they would like to be treated in labor.

It has been suggested (Price 1998) that writing a birth plan forms part of the ritual of preparing for birth in the way that knitting a layette and retiring from public life did formerly, and it certainly provides a good opportunity to focus on your feelings about the forthcoming birth and baby.

Writing a birth plan should perhaps be considered almost like a diary, as emotions and wishes can alter greatly during the course of pregnancy. Women at the end of pregnancy frequently comment how little they knew at the start, and that they did not then know what it was that they wanted and so were content to be guided by professionals. By the end, they are much more certain (although they sometimes feel they would have done things differently but find it too difficult to initiate change at that stage). It can be valuable to write a plan, even if you know your midwives well, to remind them and your partner of your wishes during labor, when you may be unable to express yourself adequately.

You may find it easier to write a birth plan from scratch rather than use one provided by the hospital, because it may be restricted, limiting you to a sort of menu of things which you are allowed. If you write a plan, it will be easier to incorporate your own wishes, although it should be kept fairly brief; seven sides of closely written script will not be easy to read and may alienate your midwife.

It is said that midwives can be antagonized by requests that they regard as normal practice; for example, no episiotomy unless absolutely necessary. However, you have no way of knowing for sure that the midwife who attends you in labor is the one who fervently believes in this policy, and it is probably better written than not. However, it is a good idea to accentuate the positive: "I would prefer . . ." rather than "Under no circumstances will I . . ." Some birth plans can read rather dictatorially and a midwife has to be high minded not to feel a bit resistant. Moreover, the nature of labor can mean that ideals are discarded in the event, and it can be harder to take if you have been very dogmatic about them.

Obviously, your wishes must be within the bounds of reality and this is where plans provide a useful point for discussion prenatally. If you rough out your plan and then discuss it with your midwife, you can find out if it is practicable, providing everything goes well. You can ask what the policy is on specific issues; it may be open to change if negotiated individually. If the hospital or staff are adamant that they cannot, or will not, provide what you want, then you have time to research other options.

If you want to change your birth plan, discuss it with your caregivers so that they are kept informed. They will find it helpful to know of your changing views. Keep your plan with you; it is likely to be most valuable if you go into labor unexpectedly and are attended by staff you do not know. You or your partner should make sure that the maternity staff read it when you are admitted, and not later.

The sort of issues you may want to include are:

- the place of birth
- pain relief
- mobility
- position of delivery
- management of third stage
- care of baby afterwards
- time together
- feeding

There will be others. Make sure that you list those which are of most importance to you, even if you think they might sound insignificant. It is just that sort of detail that a midwife may not be able to get right intuitively.

• *Relaxation* •

All prenatal classes will teach some form of relaxation technique even if it is only a simple way of using breathing to help you through contractions.

Many will spend quite a large part of the classes giving you ideas for consciously relaxing your muscles, so that you can help yourself to relieve tension at any time. Techniques of this kind have a wide application and once learned can be usefully practiced on the occasions when you find yourself getting tense and frustrated. They are especially useful in the early days of parenthood, when awareness of constant responsibility for your baby can make your prepregnancy ways of relaxing difficult or impossible.

A technique that is often suggested is known as progressive relaxation where you tense muscles and then become aware of how they feel once you remove all the tension from them and let them go. Some people feel that some residual tension may be felt in this way and that it is better just to relax from normal rather than actively tensing muscles. As with all preparation for labor, the more you do, the easier it becomes and the better able you will be to use it while your uterus is contracting powerfully. If you are able to let go and relax, the uterine muscles will be able to work without being restricted by tension.

As you become more familiar with relaxation techniques you will be able to practice them in the sorts of upright positions that are most helpful in labor: leaning over a board or ledge; sitting on a back-to-front chair; kneeling; kneeling forward over cushions, birth ball or bean bag; standing and walking; rocking hips to and fro, swaying from side to side; etc.

Relaxation Technique
You can teach yourself to relax easily by following these instructions, which are fairly universal. You may come to prefer methods taught in your prenatal class, which may be supported by a tape produced by your class facilitator, but you can start this way early in pregnancy, long before classes start.

1 Start by making sure that you are not hungry or thirsty, and empty your bladder if necessary. Make sure that you will not be interrupted; put the answering machine on if necessary.

2 Find a comfortable sitting position, supported by cushions or pillows if you wish. Put a blanket over you if you feel cold.

3 Breathe out first, then take in as much air as you need. Sigh it out gently and then breath normally. Be aware of breathing in calm and confidence, and that with each outward breath you are breathing out any tension and anxiety you may be feeling.

4 Next, become aware of different parts of your body, think about them in turn and then actively relax or release the tension within them. Start to feel your body getting heavier and spreading out a little bit more.

5 First, think about your left foot; your toes are relaxed and still, your foot is resting easily. Now your right foot; your toes are relaxed and still and resting comfortably.

6 Now, think about your ankles, roll them outwards and leave them, and move up your legs, making sure that the muscles of your calves are soft and relaxed without any tension in them.

7 Move upwards, checking your knees and thighs, making sure that they feel loose and comfortable.

8 Be aware of your pelvis. Release any tension in the hips or buttocks. When you are sure that they feel soft and loose, move up to your abdomen. Remind yourself to breathe normally and comfortably, letting all your tension go as you concentrate on the out-breath. Give your abdomen a little push out with the abdominal muscles and then relax. Don't hold the muscles in.

9 Now, concentrate on your fingers. Stretch them gently and then let them relax, curved and limp against your body. Feel your arms relaxing too, and then move up to your shoulders. Drop them, so that any tension that you feel in them melts away. Try to keep your neck long and relaxed. Move your head from side to side until it feels completely comfortable.

10 Next, concentrate on your face, let your jaw drop so that it is relaxed, feel your tongue soft and loose inside your mouth. Keep your cheeks soft and your lips apart. Close your eyes gently, let your lids rest softly on them. Make sure that your head feels heavy and that its weight is being supported by the surface that it is resting on.

11 Think about your forehead and allow it to become smooth and unfurrowed. Feel that your scalp is loose over your head, that no tension can be felt in your head, shoulders, arms, chest,

abdomen, thighs, knees, calves, ankles, or feet.

12 Listen to your calm, slow, deep breathing and relax.

13 When you feel rested and relaxed, come to by breathing in energy, breathing away any tiredness. Return to the present. Become aware of your surroundings and open your eyes.

As you practice this relaxation technique you will become increasingly aware of the sensations of your body, and practiced in the skill of allowing parts of your body to relax while other parts are working to keep you upright. As pregnancy progresses, try relaxing in the positions that you would like to use in labor, concentrating particularly on the area around your uterus. It can be helpful to rehearse relaxation and breathing techniques whenever you have Braxton-Hicks contractions or other discomfort.

Breathing in through your nose and out through your mouth slowly, concentrating on the out-breath works wonderfully for relieving pain of any kind and is a valuable way to help children to handle pain.

Although conscious relaxation is not the instinctive reaction to pain it is something which, if learned, can help you to listen to your instinct about giving birth and obey it.

The more it is practiced, the more effective it will be.

• *Massage* •

To be touched or held in labor can be very therapeutic. Several studies (Birch 1986, Rubin 1963, Lovensen 1983) have discovered that increased touch – stroking, affectionate hugs, holding, rubbing, pressure, patting – have helped women. Women who were mainly touched on the back and hands also found it useful when it included legs, feet, abdomen, arms, forehead, side, and perineum. Touch was viewed less as pain relief and more as providing a feeling of being supported by someone else, comforted and cared for, reassured and safe. Women felt encouraged by touch, and closer to and more able to rely on the person touching them. Interestingly, some women found it most helpful during transition, usually believed to be a time when women are least likely to appreciate being touched. Touch is of great value, particularly if a woman feels free to say when it is not helping.

Massage, which is a more organized form of simple touch, can help to relieve pain and tension because it relaxes muscles and induces a feeling of well-being. It is useful during pregnancy to ease aches and pains, and it can also improve the circulation and digestion, and stimulate the lymphatic system – invaluable for swollen feet, ankles, and legs.

Massage is probably the most helpful thing that a birth partner can do for a woman in labor. It will ease pain and prevent a woman from feeling isolated. It is also very therapeutic for the person giving the massage as it is something effective that he or she can do to help. It provides a very reassuring way to demonstrate love and affection and a sharing of the birth experience. It can be agonizing to watch someone you love in pain and feel that there is nothing that you can do to help. Providing massage is wonderfully soothing for the mother, but calming for fathers too. Ideally, massage should be practiced in pregnancy so that you are able to explore what is most helpful and improve technique, but it is not essential.

Massage Techniques
To give a massage, try the following – although it is vital to be guided by what a woman finds valuable. Bear in mind that this can change rapidly so that something which was appreciated may suddenly become irritating. Do not feel offended if she suddenly snaps at you – it is not intended personally.

- Make sure you are as comfortable as possible before starting. Kneel on one knee or have one foot behind the other if you are standing. Massaging for long periods is demanding and you should make it as easy for yourself as possible.
- Use talcum powder or oil to reduce friction on the skin (see pages 96–97 for massage-oil recipes for labor).
- Breath in a relaxed way, breathing from your abdomen. She will pick up your breathing rhythm.
- Rest your hands on her for thirty seconds before beginning.
- Massage toward the heart: upward from the legs, downwards from the shoulders.
- Always keep one hand on her body.
- Try to establish a rhythm so that it feels like a smooth, continuously flowing stroke.
- Vary the pressure: lighter over bones, firmer over large areas of muscle.
- Ask her to let you know if it is not helping; you need to be very responsive.
- When the mother is on all fours, support her head with one hand under her forehead and massage her back with the other.

You need to be well braced to support the weight of her head. If she relaxes into this position, you will find it heavy.

- Feet often become cold in labor, and women may twist one against the other. It can help just to hold each one firmly or to hold one foot between both hands.
- Support one foot with one hand and stroke the sole firmly with the heel of your other hand.
- Stroke up her forehead into the hairline stroking gently with one hand following the other in a rhythmic sequence. Gentle stroking round the face and jaw can be helpful too.
- Press your thumbs firmly into the center of the buttocks to relieve backache.

Other useful techniques include:
- Using both hands, stroke gently but firmly from the shoulders down to the fingertips. It can be useful just to hold the shoulders firmly but not tightly.
- Place your hands on her shoulder and massage her neck and shoulders with your thumbs, concentrating on areas that seem particularly tense.
- Massage down her back, starting at the shoulders and moving down to the base of her spine: one should follow the other in a continuous stream.
- Massage the inner or outer thighs firmly upward concentrating on the inner thigh.
- Try very light massage with fingertips around the abdomen, starting well up one side, going underneath and coming up the other side. This technique is known as effleurage – and is likely to be either welcome or irritating.

Make it clear when you are about to stop massaging by slowing the rhythm gradually and eventually stopping and then taking your hands off slowly.

• *Eating and Drinking in Labor* •

It makes sense to eat well while you can because labor uses up large amounts of energy. You may or may not feel like eating, and at some point the process of digestion slows down so that energy can be concentrated on contractions, powerfully strong muscular movements, which although they are involuntary still use up large amounts of energy. Logically it seems likely that your body would benefit from having calories to fuel this effort. If you are giving birth at home, there will be nothing to stop you eating and drinking as you wish during labor. However, this logic does not seem to apply to women giving birth in the hospital who can still, in the main, expect to be denied food and drink during labor.

It is worth looking at the reasoning behind this practice in order to see why it is done, and also to examine its relevance to giving birth today.

Why Are Food and Drink Withheld During Labor?

The reason is that a woman might require a general anesthetic for an emergency cesarean section, she might vomit food or drink while under anesthetic, and she might then inhale the vomit which would cause fatal lung failure. This is known as Mendelson's syndrome and was indeed responsible for the death of sixteen women in the years 1970–72. However, there are a number of factors which made the policy irrelevant then, and make it even more so today.

First, it is extremely unlikely that a woman will inhale vomit if she is allowed to eat and drink as she wishes in labor, but if she does inhale anything, the contents of her stomach are likely to be less acid and caustic than the contents of an "empty" stomach which contains very acidic gastric juices.

Second, although the cesarean-section rate is rising rapidly, the number of operations done under general anesthetic is decreasing fast. Nearly all are done under epidural, except for very sudden emergencies. Moreover, anesthetic technique has been much improved in the last thirty years.

Problems Linked with Starvation

A very interesting example of the way in which withholding food from laboring women can affect the outcomes of their labor was described by Leslie Ludka (1988). In a poverty-stricken, socially deprived area of the Bronx there is a hospital that models its policy on Dutch hospital services. Policy for ten years, with 20,000 births, was to allow women to eat and drink lightly, as they wished, throughout normal labor. In all those births, not one woman aspirated (inhaled) vomit.

But for a six-month period, they starved women. The results were dramatic. They had their first case of maternal aspiration in a woman who had had nothing by mouth for 36 hours. Use of synthetic oxytocin rose five-fold, instrumental delivery increased by 35 percent and cesarean-section rates increased by 38 percent. Vaginal births following a previous cesarean section fell by 37 percent and the need for intensive care of the newborn increased by 69 percent.

Fortunately, the policy was withdrawn and the health of mothers and their babies returned to the previously high norm.

Starvation is recognized as being responsible for other problems. Ketonuria, the presence of ketones in the urine of laboring women, which indicates that the body is deriving its energy directly from body fat, was conventionally treated by putting the woman on an intravenous drip containing glucose, to which Pitocin may be added because ketosis also slows the process of labor. Not surprisingly, this can cause problems of its own. But it has been suggested (Keppler 1988) that not only is some ketosis in labor normal, and therefore should not be treated except by allowing the woman to eat and drink, but that there are considerable disadvantages to administering a glucose drip. These include the risk of infection, the risk to mother and baby of giving too much sugar (hyperglycemia), which can lead to the baby producing too much insulin which may lead to the newborn baby having too little sugar (neonatal hypoglycemia) and neonatal jaundice. These potential side effects are added to the considerable discomfort of having a drip in your arm, confinement to the area where the drip-stand is placed, and the clear message that you are a patient requiring the hospital's assistance to give birth. The author suggests that as women at full-term are carrying an extra $3\frac{1}{2}$ pints of water it is unlikely that they will become dehydrated anyway, and that "partial dehydration and moderate ketosis may well be a normal and even beneficial part of labor and may be essential in protecting the brain from hypoxic damage". In this area, as in others, it seems that the body is designed to be able to give birth without drips, needles, and injections provided women are allowed to trust their instincts – in this case, to eat and drink as they wish.

Planning Ahead

When you labor at home, you can eat or drink what you please. It can be a good idea to have put something aside beforehand, and to have a range of things to choose from. Easily digested foods are often recommended, but it could be anything that you feel like.

If you intend to have your baby in the hospital, find out beforehand about the policy regarding eating and drinking. Some places allow nothing, some water or ice chips only, others drinks, and in some you may have anything. If your wishes are likely to be counter to the current policy you will need to discuss them beforehand and include them on your birth plan. It is not helpful to have a disagreement during labor, although your wishes should be paramount except in an emergency. The evidence from the Bronx suggests that depriving women of food and drink is actually harmful to them and their babies but this is not the consensus view. If you encounter a rigid non-eating policy, it may be time to think of having your baby elsewhere.

· *Clothing in Labor* ·

Nowadays, many women end up wearing nothing when they give birth – modesty being the last thing on their mind.

However, there is certainly something to be said for having something on or with you that smells reassuring and familiar, particularly in a hospital setting, and babies often find it easier to sleep when put to bed with their mother's none too clean nightie.

Women can get very hot in labor (with the exception of the feet which may become very cold) and the best things to wear are made of cotton or linen and are very loose. People often use a large man's shirt, a T-shirt, a nightie, or a maternity top; you need it to be free at the bottom if you are going to give birth while wearing it. If you are using a TENS machine it is helpful to have something to hang it on. If your waters have gone you will need elasticated pants and either a waterproof backed pad or baby's disposable diaper, to catch the liquid.

Long hair should be tied back or up – it tends to get in the way of massage and become sweaty.

· *Packing a Birth Bag* ·

Emphasis is often placed on having your bag packed and ready from 36 weeks of pregnancy. Unfortunately, this tends to create the impression that labor will be a matter of urgency, when there will be no time to lose as you swing into action and snatch it up. This will only be true for a minority of women, usually those who have already had a child. For the rest, getting a bag ready should be regarded as an opportunity to really think about the contents.

If you are having a baby in the hospital you want to take with you everything that will contribute to you feeling as comfortable and relaxed as possible. People make jokes about the amount of equipment that couples take with them, but it is not excessive when you think that you are trying to recreate the benefits of home.

It is important to have ready a bag, or at least a collection of things that you might need, even if you are having your baby at home. The air of relaxation that a home birth warrants can mean that you can be too laid back and find yourself having to scramble around for the camera just as the head is crowning. Moreover, if you do need to transfer to the hospital, you will need your things with you all the more.

Labor is a very special occasion, one which most people find exciting and feel benevolently towards. The rules of everyday living are suspended so that normal responsibilities are removed, and it should be a time when you are free to do what you want, when nearly everyone will go out of their way to help you. You will only have this labor once, so it is worthwhile to think carefully about what you can take or have, in order to make the occasion as enjoyable as possible. Indulge yourself in the preparations you make, and don't worry about what other people will think of the sort of things that you find comforting. What is important is what matters to you.

Consider everything you might need. Although it can seem quite reasonable to think that you may pick up things at the time, or on the way there, or for your partner to run home and get them, in the excitement of the moment you may forget to take them, or find that it's nighttime and all the shops are shut, or that the hospital cafeteria is not open. Moreover, when you reach a labor room, you are unlikely to want to be left by yourself. The world seems to shrink down into that room, and time and space take on a different dimension unrelated to the world outside.

Here are some suggestions including what you will need during labor and after your baby is born.

Things Needed During Labor
- Loose cotton clothing
- Cardigan
- Warm socks
- Camera or video camera and film
- Music: walkman/other
- Entertainment, puzzle, game, book
- Notepad and pen
- Calling card

- Massage oil for labor: essential oils mixed with sweet almond base oil, *and/or*
- Talcum powder for massage (baby powder is good)
- Water spray
- Hot water bottles, frozen ice packs (such as picnic coolers)
- TENS machine (this should be on before you leave for the hospital)
- Positioning aids: pillows, futon, bean bag
- Homeopathic kit
- Sponge
- Several washcloths
- Hairband/hairclips
- Perfume (although strong scents can delay breastfeeding)
- Any charm/mascot/amulet
- Flowers
- Plastic bags
- Cotton diapers
- Rubber gloves
- Bucket. The diapers can be used as hot compresses on your back, perineum, or inner thighs. Soak them in a bucket of very hot water and wring out using the gloves. You can add essential oils to the water. Diapers can also pad the bucket if you wish to squat on it.
- Electric fan: often very welcome, but in short supply in hospitals

Food and Drink
- Sandwiches and anything else; for example, fruit, dried fruit, sweets, chocolate, biscuits
- Plenty to drink: sports drinks, bottled water, fruit juice
- Thermos containing tea, coffee, or homemade soup. Particularly good for herb tea, such as raspberry leaf, chamomile, fennel
- Thermos with wide neck containing ice cubes, plain or made from raspberry leaf tea or fruit juice
- Flexible straws

Chapter Seven

POSITIONS IN LABOR

To look at the position which women naturally or instinctively adopt in labor we have to look at the past and to societies that have not been touched by Westernization. Although reports of what actually happened in labor are frustratingly few, it is reasonably clear that women delivered in a variety of different positions when they were able to choose for themselves, although they would still be guided by local custom. In Tudor and Stuart England, a popular medical book stated:

> *all women are not delivered after one fashion; for some are delivered in their bed; others sitting in a chair, some standing being supported and held up by the standers by; or else leaning upon the side of a bed, table, or chair; others kneeling being held up by the arms.*

Historians and anthropologists who have investigated the position that women choose to give birth (Engleman; Gélis) have found that the majority are either upright, kneeling, or squatting (crouching, as Gélis describes it). It is only during the last two centuries, in Western society, that the recumbent or semi-recumbent position has achieved popularity. In many places today it is still mandatory, although there is a growing realization, backed up by research, that not only are horizontal positions not what women choose but that they are also inefficient; they can prolong labor, make it more painful, can have a deleterious effect on the mother's blood pressure, and can reduce the supply of oxygen to the baby.

Adopting an Upright Position
Fortunately, evidence of physiological benefits is now available to back women's instinctive preference for an upright position so that no one now need labor lying down unless she chooses to – although the presence of a bed in a delivery room can still make a silent suggestion. Upright positions need to be defined; they are when a woman is standing, sitting, squatting, or kneeling. A horizontal position is when she is lying on her back, her side, in the lithotomy position, on her hands and knees, or in the semi-recumbent position,

which is often favored in hospitals, with the woman on her back but propped up by pillows, cushions or wedges.

The upright position during the first stage of labor has been shown to result in less severe pain, a reduced need for epidurals and other pain-relieving drugs, a better heart rate in the baby and a shorter labor. The reasons include the fact that, due to gravity, the contents of the uterus press down more efficiently on proprioceptors in the cervix and eventually the pelvic floor, which causes a surge in output of oxytocin which is responsible for the contractions of the uterus. It also helps to relax the pelvic ligaments which can be of particular importance as the baby descends through the pelvis (Young 1940).

It has been shown (Borell 1966) that the symphysis pubis can be displaced downwards by as much as 1 inch as the head comes down through the pelvis, and as much as ¾ inch upwards from the original position during the actual birth.

The pressure of the uterus in an upright position is increased so that the drive or thrust through is more efficient, and it may be better for the baby's brain as the greatest force falls on the most developed part. Laboring on one's back can reduce the mother's blood pressure and decrease the amount of oxygen available to the baby because the weight of the uterus compresses large blood vessels. Many women find lying on their back in late pregnancy very uncomfortable, or even impossible, as it makes them feel faint.

Birthing Chairs

Giving birth upright has advantages too, although not for the birth attendants who, as Pare found, will be at a physical disadvantage.

Universally, birthing chairs or stools follow a strikingly similar design: with a horseshoe or crescent shaped rim on which the mother could support her weight; a cut-away area so that her sacrum and coccyx are not under pressure and are free to move; and perhaps a sloping back and arm rest to grip during contractions. Some had a skirt to protect the parts from the dreaded drafts. Some birthing chairs could be taken apart and carried by the midwife, while others were made of willow with a high back and a built in canopy – also used for invalids.

Birthing stools and chairs may still be used today. In a 1995 study it was shown as a result of thirteen randomized, controlled trials, that women who remained upright in the second stage of labor, while they gave birth, felt less discomfort, less intolerable pain, had a shorter second stage, found bearing down easier, had

fewer assisted births (forceps, vacuum extractions and episiotomies), and fewer cesarean-section births. They had fewer perineal and vaginal tears but more labial tears and fewer wound
infections after the birth.

Women who used stools or chairs did bleed more, although it is
not clear if this is because more blood was likely to be recorded
when they were on the chair or stool or because blood is not so well
able to flow round the body when pressure is exerted on the thighs
and buttocks on a hard edge while bearing down.

The two trials where women used a soft cushion, or nothing, to
maintain their position showed no increased blood loss.

Supporting an Upright Position

It can be hard to find the energy or enthusiasm to maintain an
upright position for giving birth, especially after a long and tiring
labor. You may need reminding of the benefits – in particular that
the second stage should be shorter.

You are also likely to require some physical support. Labor
rooms rarely contain furniture that enables women to support
themselves. In other societies, women have ropes, hammocks or
bars to hold on to. In the past roller towels were used to hold on to,
and in France, women would suspend themselves between the
backs of two chairs. Although it is possible to get a bar, which will
slot into the lithotomy stirrup poles, to give a mother a way of
assisting a squatting position on the bed or to help her hang on to
it from the floor, it seems to be little used. Some hospitals supply
beanbags and mattresses so that women can lean forward over
them to rest on between contractions. It is unusual to find support
other than that provided by a chair or stool – and even these are not
commonplace.

You can, of course, use human support: either with an arm
around each supporter's neck, or with a partner supporting you
under the arms, or turning face to face and hanging from his neck,
or semi-sitting on a knee of each of two supporters. These positions
are comforting but difficult to maintain for a long time.

It is well worth finding out about the policy of the unit or practice of the midwives that you expect to help you give birth. They
may endorse an upright position for delivery, but need to be experienced in doing it. It can be hard for someone who is used to
women delivering on their backs or in a semi-sitting position, to
reorient themselves to a baby being born with its mother on hands
and knees, for example, and midwives are unlikely to encourage

you to try positions they do not feel confident about. If you feel strongly about being encouraged to be upright in labor and to give birth, you should make sure that it has been discussed well before you go into labor. It may also be necessary to remind staff when you are in labor too.

Birth Ball

A new aid to labor, which is relatively inexpensive and well worth trying, is the birth ball. This is a large, inflatable, tough, plastic ball which is big enough to lean over. It can be used during pregnancy to assist optimal fetal positioning (see page 65) and it is very versatile in labor. The birth ball can be used to replace pillows or bean bags as a support for leaning against or over, and can be used for rocking rhythmically backward and forward over (Anderson 1998). Birth balls can easily be transported to hospital deflated.

If you are considering buying one it is suggested that you get it at least a month before you are due so that you can practice using it beforehand.

· *Fetal Monitoring* ·

Your baby's heart beat will be monitored during labor to assess how well it is standing up to the stress of contractions. It can be done by several means, including:

- A Pinard stethoscope, a trumpet-like stethoscope that a caregiver presses to your abdomen and listens through directly.
- A hand-held Doppler machine, where the transducer is pressed to your abdomen and an audible and visible signal is emitted with the heart rate showing on a small screen.
- A transducer is attached to your abdomen via a belt, so the heart rate can be heard and seen, and a paper trace recording is made (Cardiotocograph or CTG).
- An electrode is attached to the baby's scalp and a similar trace printed out.

These last two methods are known as Electronic Fetal Monitoring (EFM) and may be used continuously.

The issue of fetal monitoring is of interest because of the effect that EFM methods can have on your labor and the questionable benefits to the baby.

Electronic fetal monitoring was introduced in the United States in the 1970s and its use spread rapidly so that within ten years it was used routinely. It was assumed that providing more detailed information about the baby's heart rates while its mother was in labor would lead to an improvement in outcome—the baby's health at birth in particular since fewer babies would suffer from lack of oxygen, thought to lead to brain damage and cerebral palsy and potentially, stillbirth. However, EFM was introduced without randomized, controlled testing. It has now been subjected to such trials including 58,555 pregnant women and their 59,324 babies, in the U.S., Europe, and Australia. The trials included women who were thought to be both at high and low risk of having complications in labor.

Unfortunately, the results were consistent in showing that not only did EFM fail to improve the outcomes, compared with hand-held monitoring or listening with a stethoscope, but that it resulted in a vast increase in unnecessary obstetric intervention. The only benefit to babies was a reduction in the number who had seizures after birth, but the babies with more seizures – who had not had EFM – did not go on to have cerebral palsy, one of the outcomes EFM was designed to avoid. In fact, the rate of cerebral palsy was slightly higher in the EFM group.

EFM, when used without taking blood samples from the babies, increases the cesarean-section rate by 160 percent. If used with blood sampling it is raised by 30 percent. The rate of operative delivery – that is, forceps and vacuum extraction – is increased by thirty percent.

It would be bad enough if a technique only proved to be of little benefit, but as the increase in surgical birth rates show, it can be positively harmful, not only to those women who have unnecessary cesarean sections or forceps deliveries, but to every woman because EFM is literally confining.

Belt Monitor
For a belt monitor to be used it is necessary to strap two belts quite tightly around your abdomen. Under one is the trans-ducer to pick up the baby's heartbeat, and under the other is a pressure gauge, the tocograph, which measures the strength of contractions. These are connected by leads to a machine that gives an immediate sound and digital reading as well as printing out the information on paper. The belt has to be tight to be effective and the sound and record of the heart-beat is easily lost when the baby moves so it can require constant adjustment. You have to remain still to be moni-

tored, generally for a minimum of twenty minutes, and it is usually done with a woman lying on her side or back which, as we have seen, can have a deleterious effect on labor.

Scalp Electrode
The other form of EFM is even more invasive and restricting. It involves rupturing membranes if they are intact and attaching an electrode to the leading part of the baby. This is screwed or clipped into the skin of the baby's presenting part – normally its scalp. A fluid-filled catheter can be put inside the uterus as well to register the force of the contractions. Both are connected by a lead to the monitor which gives results in the same way as the cardiotocograph. The fetal scalp monitor is very restrictive because you cannot move beyond the reach of the lead, and you are generally expected to use it until the baby is born. There is a very small risk that the electrode may be misplaced.

Interpretation and Benefits
Electronic fetal monitoring is very sensitive and picks up all signs that can be interpreted as fetal distress in a baby. However, we still find it hard to interpret fetal heart rates; so that a baby who is apparently distressed may turn out to be fine when delivered by emergency cesarean section. It may be that some signs of distress are part of a normal reaction to labor, and interpreting an EFM trace or listening to a hand-held Doppler depends on the skill and experience of the practitioner. Some obstetricians, when shown the same trace a week apart, differed in the decisions that they made on its basis – showing that it is an inexact science.

The evidence shows quite clearly that there is no overall benefit to using electronic fetal monitoring to women at low risk of complications, and that it can be positively harmful by causing unnecessary interventions. It has been estimated that 926 women would have to have an unnecessary cesarean section to prevent one case of brain damage as a result of labor (Grant 1997). (See pages 131–135 for more details on cesarean section.) It is also not proven that EFM benefits high-risk labor either, although it can be supposed that it might, and you may feel happier having it if you know your baby is at increased risk of becoming short of oxygen. There is no evidence that the routine trace done by EFM, when a woman is admitted to hospital in labor, is of any value. It is believed that listening with a Doppler is more accurate than listening in with a stethoscope, and it can be used while a woman is upright and when a woman is using a pool.

The research suggests that monitoring of a baby's heartbeat is worthwhile in order to detect abnormally fast or slow heart rates which may indicate a problem, although there is no consensus on how frequently this should be done. Hand-held monitoring is the safest method of monitoring the baby in normal labor and you would be entitled to refuse EFM on the grounds that it can do more harm than good (Thacker 1998).

• *Jeanette James* •

I was planning to have my first child, Ruby, at home but after I had been having contractions for twenty-four hours, we eventually went to the hospital because I had become very tired – even though I used to run marathons. We were also becoming concerned because it was taking so long. Because it was night-time when I went into labor, the midwife who had called suggested that I try to get some sleep, by either lying down or leaning over a bean bag. I found this incredibly painful.

In the morning, my prenatal teacher came over and we went for a walk around the Green, but it was the day before Christmas Eve and bitterly cold, and I was so tired and cold that we were forced to come inside. When we got to hospital I chose an epidural which brought instant relief, although the effects seemed to wear off more and more quickly so that I would suddenly find myself experiencing the peak of a contraction. In hindsight, I think it was a mistake that I was lying down for most of my labor. Ruby had to be delivered by vacuum extraction after two hours of pushing.

I planned for a home birth again for the next baby and went to Hypnotherapy for Birth classes, my goal being to have the baby at home and to have a positive experience. When it came to it – she was nineteen days late – I found that being upright was very helpful and the pain was much easier to deal with while I was on my feet, which I was for 98 percent of the time.

We went for a walk along the river while I was having contractions every five minutes, but they were not bothering me. After we had walked a couple of miles, Mark suggested that we get the bus back but I couldn't think why, so we walked the two miles back to the car. Once we got in the car, though, I felt my contractions so intensely that I had to ask him to stop driving while I dealt with them but also urged him to get home as quickly as possible so that I could be upright again.

Once I was on my feet once more they ceased to trouble me and I was quite confused by Mark suggesting that we should call the midwives and asked him why. He pointed out that I was having contractions every five minutes and that he felt we should let them know that I was in labor. Because I was nineteen days late I really think I'd forgotten I was ever going to go into labor.

When we called, they asked how I was coping with the pain. Because the contractions were so much easier to deal with than in my previous labor I couldn't work out how to describe how I was coping, so she asked me what setting the TENS machine was on (which I'd had on and off for a couple of days). When she heard that it was on ten, which is the maximum, she said that she had better come round. In fact, it needed a fresh battery; we got it down to five after that. Shortly after, when I was examined by the midwife, she gave me the positive news that I was a good 5 cm dilated.

The other thing that really helped was "belly breathing" which I was told about by a New Zealand midwife when I went for monitoring at the hospital. She showed me this method of pushing your tummy out while you are breathing in and pulling it while you are breathing out. Mark picked up on it and coached me throughout the labor which lasted eight hours from the time the midwife arrived; he helped me to regain the pattern when I lost concentration and it really was just brilliant. Just by breathing deeply and smoothly I could ease the incredible tight feeling I had across my tummy during contractions. This and the TENS saw me through.

Wallis was born after only four pushes, weighing just over 8½ pounds. This time, my pelvic floor was intact rather than feeling as if World War Three had been fought in it, and control started to return the next day rather than weeks later.

All in all, it was a much better experience than my first labor.

Chapter Eight

NATURAL AIDS TO PAIN RELIEF

· *Water* ·

Water has been used to ease the pain of labor for as long as women have had access to baths and hot water. It is a soothing and relaxing form of pain relief which also helps to soften perineal tissues; is available at home as well as in hospital; takes the weight off your body; and is good for first labors. Baths have long been recommended by midwives to ease pain, and birthing pools, which are increasingly popular, have the added advantage that a woman can change position easily. Privacy may be increased if a woman is literally out of reach of midwifery staff. Some women find it easier to relax and let labor take its course once they are in water. It has been found that getting into the pool before you are 5 cm dilated can stop a slow labor (although this finding has not been applied to having a bath).

However, unless a pool is plumbed into a maternity unit, obtaining a pool for labor and possibly birth takes quite a lot of organization and has become subject to rules and regulations which do not seem to apply to baths. There are various considerations that need to be taken into account if you want to use a birthing pool, either at home or in the hospital.

If you are planning to use a pool installed in the hospital, you should consider what you will do if it is being used by someone else at the time you need it. Other drawbacks can include the fact that a pool hired for home use can take a couple of hours to fill which may not be soon enough, especially if it is not your first baby. You may not be able to use the pool if the baby shows signs of distress while you are in labor, or if complications arise in late pregnancy, and you may simply find that when you are actually in labor you don't want to be in water after all, or that you instinctively get out for the birth. You cannot stand upright and be in water unless you labor in a swimming pool.

However, water birth is perfectly possible to arrange and is increasingly offered in maternity units. If it is available, you need to book it, and may have to pay for the use of a disposable liner. Some birthing centers or hospitals are happy for you to come in and set up a privately hired pool by arrangement. If your caregiver refuses to allow this, or if you would prefer to have your baby at home anyway, you will need to plan a home birth. It is important to have a midwife who is familiar with water births, not only for the sake of you and your baby, but in order that she feels confident too.

Birth under water is safe providing the baby is brought to the surface within a few minutes of delivery. He or she is in amniotic fluid until that time and will receive oxygen via the placenta and umbilical cord until making contact with air and taking the first breath. However, some midwives are uneasy about the prospect and will encourage a woman to get out of the pool in the moment of birth. Some units that seem to offer water birth have few births that actually take place in water. Some units have pools, but discourage their use, so it is worth finding out about the number of actual water births taking place in a unit or at home.

Some of the practical considerations involved in organizing the rental of a birth pool include:

- Cost: It is worth comparing prices, rental terms, type of pool, ease of transport. You may have to buy a pool liner as well. You may want to consider installing a big, permanent bath instead.
- Type of pool: If possible, try out the different kinds, as some may be too cramped if you are taller than about 5 feet, 4 inches. Some are easier to put up than others. Well-padded pools are more comfortable.
- Floor: You will need a strong floor to withstand the weight of water, which may be as much as 200 gallons.
- Space: You should have space beside the pool for birth to take place outside it, if necessary.
- Heating and Electricity: You will have to check arrangements for heating the pool and have the installation assessed for safety by an electrician. Current breaker switches may need to be installed.

Other things to consider:

- Temperature. The pool should be around 100.4°F in the earlier part of the labor. If it is hotter it is considered that a mother may suffer from heat exhaustion and have insufficient energy for labor.
- Rehearsal. It is a good idea to have a dress rehearsal before labor starts, to work out all the logistics, to see how long the pool takes

to fill, and so forth. You may find that you would like to invite a friend to be present to provide extra help at the birth.

· *Deborah Pentesco-Gilbert* ·

I was originally planning to have my first child in a large London maternity hospital but I didn't feel right about it, even though I couldn't really explain why. I wanted to labor in the pool and have as little intervention as possible. Although I felt that people might think me a bit hysterical or picky, I decided to change. I found that it was hard, because I didn't know where to change to or who to explain my feelings to. I eventually planned for another hospital, only to find that they were over-booked and couldn't take me. I looked at another that didn't feel right at all and then someone suggested the West Middlesex and we went on one of their Sunday-afternoon tours.

I was impressed by the midwife who showed us round who was bubbly and relaxed and offered us a cup of tea. I felt for the first time that this was somewhere I would be cared for. They suggested that I come back and discuss the reasons for changing and said it was possible to transfer myself rather than going through my doctor. They put no pressure on me but were very open and communicative and we talked for nearly two hours.

It was only three weeks before I was due; I booked there and then and found that I felt much more confident about the birth, and that I knew I would feel OK about going to hospital rather than fearing it. I felt that they were quite happy to support me to do things the way I wanted; their only concern was to make sure that what I wanted was possible. It was pot-luck as to whether the pool would be available, and not all the midwives were trained to assist at water births, so I could not be guaranteed the opportunity to labor in water. I didn't actually plan to give birth in a pool.

I went into labor a few days past my due date although I find it hard to say exactly when. I had a show on Saturday night which continued through Sunday. On Monday I had what felt like strong period pain but because the pain was at the front, and I had been expecting back pain, I didn't think it was labor. I found the most comfortable place to be was on the toilet, so I spent much of Monday sitting there and reading a book.

By seven in the evening I found that I wanted to breathe out and moan a bit to release the tension. By then the pain was still like period pain but stronger than I had ever felt. The contractions continued and for the next two hours I walked about our landing and leaned over our bannisters during contractions.

By nine, we decided that this probably was it and so dimmed the lights, turned on the music and Michael put the TENS on. That really brought relief from it. I still knew when I was having contractions but it subdued them and made them feel as if they were somewhere else. It meant that I didn't have to walk around so much and I was more able to talk to Michael. I felt better, and we were able to watch television for an hour. Then between eleven and twelve it picked up speed. By midnight contractions were coming every three minutes and Michael thought we should go in. I was convinced that we would be sent home because it wasn't hurting enough, but Michael rang and they asked us to come in.

In fact, I'm glad we went in then because I found the car journey very difficult because I didn't want to sit down. I knelt on the front seat looking out through the back window and we sped through the red lights. When we got there I was glad to be upright again and not at all keen to lie down to be monitored. We reached a compromise with the student doctor holding the monitor in place while I moved around. It turned out that I was 4 cm dilated. I wanted to kiss the midwife because it meant that we didn't have to go back home, although I also felt alarm at the thought that this was really going to happen.

The pool was free about half an hour after we got there, and had to be refilled, so that I was able to get in at about 1:30 A.M. I was quite scared to take the TENS off and so tried turning it right down for a couple of contractions. Then I said OK, they took it off, and I got in. The relief was instant; I'm not sure whether it was because it eased contractions or because it relieved the weight of the baby, but I found that I was able to talk to Michael again which had become quite hard. I found it wonderful to be weightless and to be able to change positions without having to struggle or ask someone to help me. I spent a lot of time on all fours but also floated on my front holding on to the edge like a little kid during contractions. I also felt protected in the water – I didn't want to be touched – and it helped to have Michael breathing with me.

At about 4 P.M. I found that I was starting to push with contractions, and they found I was fully dilated, so topped up the hot water and said that I could push. I was pushing on all fours which was fine, but the midwife asked me to turn so that I was alternately floating and squatting, supported by Michael and the student midwife on each side, gripping their hands tightly. I found the water really helpful because I could tilt my pelvis back and forward so easily.

I had been making a lot of noise – anyone outside must have thought they were killing me – and I found it easier to be uninhibited about it in the water. Being able to make a noise was really helpful. However, the midwife advised me to use the energy to help push him out. I didn't find that it hurt as much as I had thought: crowning felt like tingling or stretching like pulling out the corners of your mouth as they had said in class. I found it really bizarre to think that they could see part of his head, but that we had to wait for the next contraction to see the rest. With a few pushes Benjamin catapulted out into the water.

The midwife gently lifted him up on to me and we kept his body in the water until the cord stopped pulsating, which took ten to fifteen minutes. After that, Benjamin was taken out to have his fingers and toes counted and the placenta followed quite quickly after he was put to the breast.

We looked in fascination at the placenta and then the midwife asked to see if I needed any stitches. I found this prospect quite terrifying and happily accepted some pain relief. They said I had a second degree tear, which I said I didn't want stitched. They got a second opinion, and then agreed, provided they kept an eye on it and I didn't bleed more heavily. As it happened, I took Arnica and it healed well without them.

Then I had the best cup of tea of my life and they turned down the lights and left us together for about an hour. We were discharged the next day.

It was the most beautiful experience and I'm sure that it would not have gone that way if I had not felt comfortable about where I was. It was well worth the effort of changing my plans. I feel quite blessed.

• *Music* •

Music has been used as an aid to relieving pain in dentistry where it has been found (Standley 1986) that auditory stimuli may directly suppress pain neurologically. Obviously it has been used for enjoyment: listening; dancing; or to increase stamina and timing as in marching. However the research on its value in actual labor rather than experimental laboratory conditions is limited, although it has been described in detail in varous research papers.

One trial involving pain – induced by suspending a Plexiglass wedge from the left index finger – found that easy listening, rather than rock music or the patient's own choice, worked best to reduce the level of pain reported by the subjects. Another trial (Turk & Gaest 1979) found that music – the Canon in D, the Suite in B flat, and Suite in G by Pachelbel – combined with imagery their subjects invoked for themselves was most helpful in reducing pain under laboratory conditions.

Clearly, artificial pain induction is nothing like labor because you can stop it at any point and it does not affect as large an area of the body. However, using a Walkman during labor can help cut out extraneous noise, help you to visualize yourself elsewhere and may increase your stamina. Common sense would seem to dictate that music you like best will be most helpful, combined with imagining yourself in pleasant surroundings.

It certainly seems as though using the music beforehand in several rehearsals – perhaps using painful stimuli such as holding an ice cube in both hands – could increase the potential benefit. There is evidence to show that rehearsal of this kind can reduce pain in labor. (Johnson J 1973, Johnson J 1978).

If you are musically inclined or merely would like to be able to shut out the sounds of the delivery room it seems worthwhile trying music as a safe and economical way of helping to reduce the awareness of labor pain.

• *Herbal Medicines* •

Until comparatively recently, herbs and alcohol preparations from plants were the only pharmacological way of alleviating the pain of labor. Although there is far less information on the particular herbs women used to relieve pain, rather than what they used to prevent or procure miscarriage and what they used postpartum, there is sufficient evidence to show how prevalent herbal use was. Even today the strongest painkillers, such as morphine, are derived from plants.

In the majority of the world's cultures, plants are used to enhance health and treat illness. The World Health Organization estimates that 75 percent of the world's population treats themselves in this way. Herbs are of particular interest because, like many long-standing therapies, they are capable of treating a far wider range of ill health or imbalances than western medicine and the risks of adverse side effects are considerably less. Many modern pharmaceuticals are plant-based but their active ingredients have been isolated and extracted in order to treat symptoms rather than the whole person and the cause of the symptoms.

Herbs which are unprocessed and used as flowers, leaves, bark, or roots, contain elements within themselves to protect users from the harm that might result from taking an extracted constituent. For example, dandelion, which is an effective and well-known diuretic, also contains potassium. Diuretic drugs have to have potassium added to them to prevent potassium deficiency which otherwise occurs as a result of diuretic drug therapy.

Historical evidence suggests that women healers and midwives were very familiar with herbs and their actions for use in childbirth and afterwards and these women were known to grow specific plants in the garden to help in their work.

Although there is only limited information about the remedies that women took to ease pain and accelerate slow or difficult labor, the names of some herbs do recur repeatedly, throughout various cultures, suggesting that they were useful. For example *Mitchella repens* – also known as partridge berry or squaw root – was made into a tea by Cherokee Indians who drank it for weeks before having a baby to hasten childbirth and make labor easier. The Shakers also used bethroot or birthroot (*Trillium oratum*), one of several species of birthroot, to ease the pain of childbirth, as well as using it as an antiseptic, astringent, and specific uterine tonic.

Preparing Herbs
There are several different ways of taking herbs, depending on whether they are fresh or dried. They can be bought in liquid form as fluid extracts or tinctures, or may be bought as dried herbs which can be made into teas or decoctions. Herbs are sometimes available in tablet form; dried and powdered herbs can be put into

capsules or made into pastes and poultices. To make a tea put 1 teaspoon of dried herb or 3 teaspoons of fresh into a teapot and pour on a cup of boiling mineral water. Allow to stand, covered, for fifteen minutes and then strain and drink it while it is still warm.

Hard and woody parts of an herb, such as roots and stems, need to be boiled to release their properties. Chop or crush the plant as much as possible before adding 1 ounce dry or 3 ounces fresh herb to 1 pint of water in a stainless steel or enamel saucepan and bringing to the boil. Simmer for fifteen minutes and then allow it to infuse off the heat before straining and drinking while still warm.

Raspberry Leaf Tea

Raspberry leaf has been taken traditionally to help women have an easier labor. It tones the uterus and is a source of iron and vitamin C. Many women have found it effective. It is made by adding a cup of boiling water to 2 teaspoons of dried leaves and allowing it to stand, covered, for fifteen minutes before straining and drinking. It can be combined with equal amounts of *Mitchella repens*. Take one cup per day throughout pregnancy or three cups a day for the last three months.

Pain-Relieving Herbs for Use Today

The number of herbs that are currently recommended for pain relief in labor, is modest, compared with those used in years gone by. Their purpose is to relieve pain and tension rather than to accelerate labor, which was the purpose of many of the herbs that used to be used in childbirth. However, the consensus is that the following are safe to take and should definitely help to relieve pain and reduce spasms.

The disadvantage of taking herbal teas in labor is that you may not be able to cope with the fluid as your digestive system slows. You may feel sick anyway. If you feel unable to sip them in water, tinctures can be taken as drops under the tongue and will act quickly. Essential oils of plants (see page 95) are useful in this situation as their properties can be dispersed into the bloodstream via massage and bypass the digestive system altogether.

Skullcap   This antispasmodic relaxes the muscles, prevents spasms, and acts as a tonic to the nervous system. It mixes well with blue cohosh, another antispasmodic that stimulates the uterus.

Take 3 to 8 drops in water. This can be repeated, but beware of its sedative effect.

Motherwort This herb is clearly specifically for mothers, and is good for the early part of a regular labor. It is a uterine stimulant, and can also be useful after giving birth to restore the uterus and reduce the risk of postpartum bleeding.

Take 5 drops of tincture in a glass of water – it works within thirty minutes and fades over 1 to 3 hours. Repeat as needed.

St. John's Wort This is useful for controlling anxiety and spasms in the back, side, and uterus.

Take 25 to 30 drops in a glass of water. Combines with skullcap.

Wild Yam Good for women who are nervous.

Compresses
A compress can be made by putting either fresh and bruised or dried and soaked herbs into a cloth, folding it over, and holding in place on the skin. Alternatively, a compress can be made by dipping the cloth into a strong infusion or decoction of an herb or by adding herbal tincture to water. The liquid can be either hot or cold and the soaked cloth is held in place until it is cooler, becomes warm, or dries out – and then the process is repeated.

Compresses of the essential oil of clary sage over the pubic bone can relieve pain particularly well. If the idea of using a compress appeals to you, have several cloths ready for use. The others can be cooling or heating while one is being applied. You can put them on the small of your back, around your head, on your wrists or inner thighs or perineum as necessary.

Herbs That Should Be Avoided in Pregnancy
Aloe vera, autumn crocus, barberry, broom, juniper, pennyroyal, poke root, parsley, southernwood, tansy, thuja, wormwood, feverfew, sassafras.

Goldenseal should not be taken during pregnancy, although it is useful for stimulating contractions in labor.

• *Aromatherapy* •

Essential oils and other smells or scents have long been used in labor to encourage the woman and induce the child to emerge.

Essential Oils from Plants

Nowadays the effects that oil distilled from plants can have on the body are more clearly defined and it is appreciated that they have pharmacological, physiological and psychological modes of action. An essential oil can effect chemical changes within the body and reacts with hormones and enzymes. It also acts physiologically by bringing about changes within the body: stimulating, sedating and so on. Its psychological effect occurs when a person reacts to its smell.

Various different combinations of oils are described as refreshing, uplifting, soothing, harmonizing, sensual, detoxifying, or good for aches and pains.

Not all plants yield essential oils, which are regarded as their lifeblood and their defense against disease. Some release much more than others, which partly explains the difference in price. For example it takes nearly half a ton of rose petals and two million jasmine flowers to make 100 grams of their oil. More information about the oils can be found in Julia Lawless's *The Encyclopaedia of Essential Oils* (see Suggested Reading, page 147).

Oils are prepared either by distillation or by the application of pressure as with citrus fruits. Distillation is achieved by means of steam, water, or solvents.

Aromatherapy can be wonderfully relaxing in pregnancy. It involves carefully massaging one or more essential oils in a carrier base oil, into the skin. It can also be used therapeutically to relieve backache, swollen legs, indigestion, heartburn, nausea and vomiting, stretch marks, constipation, hemorrhoids, varicose veins, cramps, and exhaustion. Consult a qualified aromatherapist for help with these conditions or just to gain an opportunity to relax.

An aromatherapist would be happy to mix a blend of oils to help relieve pain and tension in labor, or you could make one up yourself. The oils have been chosen for their physiological effects on the woman in labor, but it is often noted that their application has a beneficial effect on partners, midwives and any one else who enters the birthing room as the smell uplifts their spirits too.

It can be useful to get used to using the oils described on the next pages during later pregnancy – apart from clary sage and jasmine, which should not be used in pregnancy, only labor – so that the limbic part of your brain (which is where emotional and autonomic responses originate) associates the smell with a time when you were not in pain and feeling safe and relaxed at home.

When you buy essential oils for home use it is important to make sure that they are 100 percent pure as some of those that are widely available are diluted with a base oil. The difference is that almost all pure essential oils, when dropped on paper, will eventually evaporate, whereas ones diluted with a base oil will leave an oily stain.

There are various ways of using the essential oils but apart from tea tree, lavender, eucalyptus, and chamomile oils, they should be used in a carrier or base oil otherwise they may irritate your skin.

How to Use Aromatherapy Oils

Bath   Make a 6 percent blend by adding 6 drops of essential oil to a 5 ml teaspoonful of base, which can either be full-cream milk or vodka. This disperses the oil, which might otherwise sting or irritate.

If your bathtub is acrylic or fiberglass you should wipe the oil off afterward.

Massage oil

- 3 to 5 drops in 5 ml teaspoon of base oil
- 1 to 25 drops in 25 ml base oil
- 20 to 60 drops to 100 ml base oil

Use oil such as sweet almond or grapeseed as a base and ask your partner to massage it in. This will feel pleasant and ensure that the oils are absorbed into the bloodstream.

Compresses   Add a few drops of essential oil to a bowl of very hot or ice cold water, dip in a washcloth or cotton diaper, squeeze it out, and apply it to the affected area. Allow to cool or warm and repeat. Rubber gloves may be needed if the process is likely to be needed often, as in labor.

Vaporization   Add a few drops of oil to a bowl of warm water or warm a little oil in a special burner or a metal ring, which you can buy and place on a bulb in a lamp. Check with the hospital first if you want to take a burner into a maternity unit. Alternatively, you can put a drop of oil on the edge of your handkerchief or the corner of a pillowcase, so that you can benefit from an essential oil day or night.

Oils for Labor

There are essential oils that are recognized as being especially beneficial for women in labor for their properties of toning the uterus and encouraging contractions, their ability to reduce pain and relieve tension, to encourage deep breathing, to relieve spasm, and to diminish fear and anxiety and enhance a feeling of well-being. They include:

Clove Bud Oil Try adding a couple of drops of clove oil to a warm bath at the beginning of labor. Clove is a pain reliever that has a traditional use in childbirth. It is a stimulant and antispasmodic.

Rose Antidepressant, sedative, and a uterine tonic. It encourages deep and calm breathing.

Clary Sage A pain reliever that is specific for labor pain. It should not be used during pregnancy but is very valuable in labor. It is an antidepressant, an antispasmodic, a nervine (strengthens and tones the nervous system), and a sedative.

It has a great reputation for relieving pain when used in a hot compress placed above the pubic bone.

Neroli (Flower of Bitter Orange) Add two drops to a tissue and inhale to reduce fear, apprehension, or anxiety. It is an antispasmodic, a mild hypnotic, a stimulant, and a cardiac and circulatory tonic, of which it has been said "it will warm the womb and facilitate the birth". It also encourages deep, calm, rhythmic breathing.

Jasmine Known as a parturient (aiding childbirth). An analgesic and antispasmodic, it strengthens contractions, calms, and energizes.

Lavender Increases the strength of contractions and reduces the feeling of panic. Lavendar is analgesic, antidepressant, and sedative. It has been prescribed historically for "lack of nerve power".

Geranium An uplifting, balancing stimulant and antidepressant. It is also antiinflammatory and antihemorrhagic.

Ylang Ylang This oil (if you like it; some people do not) is a soothing antidepressant that has a regulating effect on cardiac and respiratory rhythm.

Cinnamon leaf Contractions may be stimulated by cinnamon leaf oil; it is an antispasmodic and a circulatory, cardiac, and respiratory stimulant.

Essential oils that should be avoided in pregnancy:
Ajowan, aniseed, basil, bay, birch, bitter almond, boldo, buchu,
camphor, clary sage, clove, cornmint, fennel (all types), horseradish,
hyssop, jasmine, lavender, cotton, *Lavendula stoechas*, mugwort,
mustard, myrrh, oregano, parsley seed, pennyroyal, plecanthrus,
rue, *Salvia officinalis*, sassafras, savin, savory, star aniseed, tansy,
tarragon, thuja, thyme (thymol type), wintergreen, wormseed,
wormwood.

• *Homeopathy* •

Homeopathic remedies can help to relieve pain in labor, but are tai-
lored to fit particular feelings, sensations, or moods and act on
them. If you would like to use homeopathy during labor, it can be
helpful to have someone with you in charge of a range of remedies.
They can be objective, observe you and ask how you are feeling,
and select the most appropriate treatment for you at that time.
Labor is regarded as an acute condition in homeopathic terms and
so tablets may be given frequently, depending on your response.

If you are not familiar with homeopathy, the theory behind it can
seem paradoxical and hard to believe because in Western medicine
the effect of a drug is increased the more that you take.
Homeopathic remedies are extremely dilute and safe for pregnancy.
Paradoxically, the more they are diluted, the more powerful they
become.

Principles of Homeopathy
The principle of homeopathy was discovered by a German, Samuel
Hahnemann, in 1796. He found that when he gave minute doses of
drugs that caused symptoms similar to an illness, it actually cured
the condition. For example, the plant that, when given to a healthy
person, would result in them having symptoms identical to malaria
could, when very much diluted, cure someone who had malaria.
This established the principle behind homeopathy which is "let like
be cured by like". The symptoms of an illness are regarded as the
body's reaction in its attempt to overcome the disease; homeopathic remedies strengthen the reaction and so help the body to heal
itself.

To benefit from homeopathy ordinarily, you would need to visit
a homeopath who will take a detailed case history and want to find
out a lot about you—not only about the problems that you are expe-

riencing currently but also about you, your personality, likes and dislikes, what makes you feel better or worse, how you relate to events and so on—before he or she would prescribe a remedy. This will be fitted to you as an individual. The treatment is for you rather than the symptom. For example, ten people with an identical cold who consulted a homeopath would each be given a different remedy.

Types of Remedies
Although it is possible to buy remedies over the counter to treat yourself for things such as insomnia or gastric upset, you generally need a proper consultation for serious or long-standing conditions. A homeopath has a knowledge of, and access to, a far wider range of remedies than a shop (there are more than 2,000) and can prescribe different potencies. The remedies that are available in shops are generally those in the lower potencies that work on a physical rather than emotional level. If the remedy fails to work it is said to be because the wrong one has been chosen.

The remedies are available in different strengths, and those that are the most dilute are the most powerful. The remedies are largely prepared from plants, although they can also be made from animal material such as cuttlefish; and from minerals that are generally regarded as inert, such as sand or gold.

They are prepared by serial dilution from a mother tincture. A tincture is made by preparing original material with water. A drop of the tincture is taken out and diluted with nine or ninety-nine drops of the diluting medium, depending on whether the potency is to be decimal (x) or contesimal (c). The mixture is shaken vigorously or "succussed", and then one drop from that tincture is taken and diluted again in the same ratio. The first dilution becomes 1c or 1x, the second 2c or 2x, and so on. The potency which is generally available over the counter is 6c and this is the potency most suitable for self-administration. The c is often omitted so that the remedy might appear as Arnica 6, for example.

The remedies come in a variety of forms; usually small hard tablets, they can also be powders, drops, soft tablets, small round pills, and tiny granules.

Taking the Remedies
Only one remedy should be taken at a time. If it fails to work after four doses another remedy should be chosen. For general use, take

one tablet three times a day for two to three days. In acute conditions, you may take a tablet six times a day, and in very painful conditions, such as earache, you may need to dose yourself as often as every fifteen minutes.

If you consult a homeopath you may find that you are prescribed fewer remedies at a higher potency. He or she may only give one or two and then wait for some days to see how you are affected by it. It is not uncommon for the illness that you want treated to appear to get worse before it gets better, and that when it improves the symptoms will go in reverse order to that in which they appeared, and from above to below, from within to without and from more vital to less vital organs.

The remedies, which are pleasant to taste, are put under the tongue and allowed to dissolve, which can take some time. It is important to take them in what is known as a "clean mouth"; that is, you should not have anything to eat or drink for the half hour before or after taking the remedy. Remedies can also be taken in warm water, and this is especially suitable for acute conditions when doses need to be taken frequently. Crush two tablets or dissolve them in a glass of warm water.

You should also avoid tea, coffee, or peppermint while you are taking homeopathic remedies because they may act as antidotes and prevent the remedy from working. Essential oils of black pepper, camphor, eucalyptus, and the mints are thought to have the same effect and should be avoided as well.

When you start to improve, increase the interval between the doses until improvement is established and then stop.

Sometimes the remedy will seem to make the condition worse (known as an aggravation). If this happens stop taking it altogether. This will probably be followed by a big improvement in your condition. You should only take it again if the symptoms recur.

The medicines are sensitive and can easily become contaminated so they must be stored in a cool dark place well away from strong smells. They should be kept in their original containers, and not touched by hand. To take one, tip some pills out into the lid and tip back those that are not needed. Then tip the remaining tablet into your mouth. If you drop one do not put it back into the bottle.

Homeopathy for Labor

The ideal way to use homeopathy in labor would be to have a trained homeopath with you. Some midwives are qualified homeopaths too and its use is growing in the maternity services but is not currently widespread. Many homeopaths would like to attend birth so it is worth asking if you have already established a relationship with one, but it may not be possible.

However, it is possible to buy homeopathic birth kits that may be used successfully by sensitive and observant birth partners. In general, they include remedies at the 200c potency as labor is a high-energy condition where the stimulus provided by the remedy may be used up quickly and may need to be repeated frequently, perhaps every fifteen minutes, or even more often.

Caulophyllum 200 Give this when contractions are ineffective or the cervix is too rigid to open. Use it when contractions are sharp and spasmodic, and the mother is exhausted, weak, and sensitive to cold.

Pulsatilla 200 This should be given when contractions begin and then stop and are ineffective. The mother is weepy, thirstless, needs attention and air, and may be begging for help. It can be useful for turning a malpositioned baby.

Kali Carbonicum 30 Give this for pains in the back, buttocks, and thighs or when the mother wants her back pressed hard. She may be sweaty, weak, anxious, or irritable, or may have a headache. This remedy may need to be repeated frequently.

Chamomilla 200 Give this when the mother is angry and irritable, and unable to bear the contractions or an examination. She may kick, swear, or strike someone. Contractions can seem to be forcing the baby up, rather than down, and she may have pain in her thighs.

Cimicifuga 200 The mother is frightened and despairing and feels out of control. She is restless and talkative. Contractions may be better if she lies on her left side.

Sepia 200 Offer this if labor is sluggish and the mother is weepy and irritable or indifferent. She may be snappy with her partner although she regrets it and feels worn out.

Aconite 30 This may be useful for both mothers or fathers who feel very fearful during the labor.

Postpartum hemorrhage
First choice: Ipecac 200
Second choice: Arnica 200

After the Birth
Aconite 30 Give this to the baby if it is shocked, blue, or unable to urinate. Give 3 to 4 doses in the first twenty-four hours of its life.

Staphisagria This is good for resentment if you feel things were done against your wishes.

Rescue Remedy
This is not a homeopathic remedy but a combination of five of Dr. Bach's flower remedies that have been found very useful to treat negative states of the mind. Each one is derived from a flower that has been floated on water in a glass bowl in full sunshine. The water is preserved in brandy and bottled.

Rescue Remedy contains Star of Bethlehem, Rock Rose, Impatiens, Cherry Plum, and Clematis. It is extremely useful in cases of mental and physical shock, terror, panic, or trauma. Take 4 drops in water if possible or put it on the lips and on the pulse points on the wrists and behind the ears.

Many families have found Rescue Remedy taken throughout labor in a glass of water (2 drops per glass) helped to sustain them and see both partners through.

• *Debra Corcoran* •

I had a planned cesarean section for my third baby because she was a footling breech. I was not looking forward to it and would have preferred to have it under general anesthetic, but they explained that it would be harder both for me and the baby to recover from, and that I might feel groggy for days and lose the first breast-feeding opportunity.

Although I would not like to go through it again, I did find taking Rescue Remedy helped me, though the effect was short-lived. It helped me to get through it and gave me something to hang on to. I think I might have jumped off the table and run away without it.

I also used Arnica successfully. One of the midwives had been very much in favor of it during our prenatal sessions and luckily she was on duty at the time and encouraged me to go on using it. I took an Arnica 200 about half an hour before the operation and another as soon as I was able to afterward. I had three separate comments on its effect. The first was from the doctor who checked me before the stitches were taken out, who asked: "Are you sure it is only three days? It's incredibly neat. It looks as though it is much farther on than it should be." The following day, the midwife who actually removed the stitches told me that she had taken out several already that morning and that mine were much better healed than any of the others. Later, when it was hurting, another midwife who looked at it said: "You do realize that you are meant to have bruising and you've got none at all!"

I was also surprised to find that I was able to turn down the offer of painkillers on a couple of occasions, which isn't my style, but I found that I didn't need them.

• *Reflexology* •

Reflexology is an ancient system of medicine that has been rediscovered in this century and is growing in popularity. It is based on the same principles as acupuncture and shiatsu (acupressure) because its practitioners believe that placing pressure or applying needles to one part of the body can relieve symptoms felt in another area. Each area of your body is reflected in a specific area of the foot, and ill health or disturbance of any particular part of the body can be described by careful examination of the area of the foot which represents it. Gentle and safe massage of the foot, concentrating on the areas where imbalance is apparent, can assist the body to heal itself.

It is less well known that the hands reflect the areas of the body too, and it is possible to treat people through gentle massage of their hands. This can be useful when treating oneself, and during labor when you may well be on your feet. Having your hand held is comforting in itself. It allows more closeness and can be done while the mother is in any position, even in a pool.

Many people find reflexology treatment particularly soothing and relaxing and it can be very beneficial during pregnancy to relieve discomfort, sickness, constipation, hemorrhoids, backache, swollen ankles, heartburn, headache, etc. It is especially helpful for women who feel anxious about giving birth and for those who have difficulty in sleeping.

If you have established a good relationship with a reflexologist you may want to invite her/him to be with you in labor. Although most reflexologists would be delighted to be asked, attending a birth presents practical difficulties for working therapists so you may need to search for a therapist who can accommodate your request.

Reflexology is a skill that more midwives are acquiring and it is worth finding out if there are any qualified reflexologists among the midwives available to you. There are certain areas of treatment for labor which are best left to those who are qualified to practice it. There are, however, techniques that can usefully be done by any birth supporter, which will help to relax you, ease the pain and tension, and encourage efficient labor. They must all be done with great gentleness, mainly on the hands.

Hands

To encourage deep relaxation, improve breathing, and provide support, your partner should take your outstretched hand with it's fingers gently curved toward you. He or she should then follow your middle finger down to your palm to the point, just below the fleshy pad at the top of the palm, where there is a slight dip. Then, watching the rhythm of your breathing, he or she should apply gentle thumb pressure at the same time as you breath in. Hold the breath for a while, and as you let it go, your partner should release the pressure. This should be repeated for three to four breaths on each hand.

To Relieve Stress and Tension   Holding your hand in his, your partner should massage gently around the base of your thumb on each hand with emphasis on the area of the crease of the joint. This helps to calm the brain and will ease tension around the shoulders and neck, which are liable to tense in painful or stressful situations.

Slow Labor   Although there is nothing particularly wrong with slow labor, if you are able to keep busy and active, there may come a point when you get fed up with it, especially if contractions prevent you from sleeping. If staff are growing impatient and talking of Pitocin drips you may want to try reflexology techniques to get labor under way. (See also pages 109–111 for other ways in which you can help to speed up labor.)

You can stimulate the pituitary gland by putting gentle pressure on the middle of the whole of your thumb.

Get your partner or midwife to rub each hand vigorously between the palms of their hands for two minutes. You can also try massaging around both your wrists briskly for a short time.

Feet

Although it is important to be upright and mobile during labor to encourage contractions that are more efficient and less painful, there may be times when you need a break and it can be soothing and comforting to have your foot massaged. Feet can get very cold in labor because energy is concentrated on contractions, and you may enjoy having them simply held firmly and warmed. Your partner can also gently massage around the area of the heels – around the ankle bone and between the ankle bone and heel on both sides of each foot.

Holding the foot in one hand gently curve the three middle fingers of the other hand, and follow the bony curve of the inside of the foot from the toe to the heel. Gradually move the fingers along, slightly lifting each portion of skin with the tips of the fingers. The pressure required is said to be no greater than that which would bruise a cranberry.

The area where the underside of the big toe follows the foot corresponds to the neck muscles (as in the thumb) and may benefit from extra attention.

Reflexology After the Birth

Reflexology may be useful afterward; it can help with a retained placenta, pain as a result of episiotomy or tears, afterpains, backache, headache (especially from breast-feeding), and postpartum depression. It can also help with engorgement and encourage a good supply of milk.

· Acupuncture ·

Acupuncture can be used very successfully, not only for pain relief during labor, but in turning breech or malpositioned babies and in inducing labor. Acupuncture involving needles in the body can restrict mobility in labor, and the use of ear points, or auricular acupuncture, is preferable. A few maternity units have midwives trained in acupuncture, but even they are not available twenty-four hours a day. In many units the TENS machine (see page 111) acts as a substitute, as the lower electrodes cover acupuncture points and TENS, like acupuncture, provides safe, drug-free pain relief.

Acupuncture is very valuable in improving health of women in pregnancy and has particular appeal because not only is the scope of its action greater than that of conventional medicine – and it can help with hemorrhoids, constipation, nausea and vomiting, headaches, severe itching, etc – but it does not involve taking anything which could potentially harm the baby. If you are lucky enough to have an acupuncturist who is able and willing to attend the birth, you may also benefit from his or her ability to speed labor, and reduce nausea as well as pain.

The Principles of Acupuncture

Acupuncture is a complete system of medicine which was developed in China over 5,000 years ago. It is based on the theory that the body is governed by two opposing parts: yin and yang. Yin is drab, cold, dark, and female. Yang is hot, stimulating, male, and related to the sun. In good health yin and yang are perfectly balanced, but in illness this balance is disturbed. If a particular organ is too yang, it is seen as being overactive, heat generating, and out of control. If it is too yin it will be sluggish, static, and full of waste. An acupuncturist can detect the balance of your body by observing you, your color and smell, and your tongue. He or she will take a full history from you and then feel the pulses on your wrists. Chinese medicine identifies fourteen separate pulses, and each one can tell the practitioner a bit about imbalances within your body.

The Chinese believe that the organs of the body are connected by invisible pathways of energy – known as meridians – so that illness in a particular organ may cause pain to be felt in another place along the meridian. Illness is thought to be caused by a blockage of the energy that should be flowing along these channels; insertion of the acupuncture needles removes the obstruction and allows energy to flow freely again.

When you have an acupuncture treatment the acupuncturist will insert needles into different parts of your body and leave them for thirty to sixty minutes. It only hurts briefly, just as the needles are inserted. Sometimes the acupuncturist may rotate the needles or send a weak electrical current through them. Heat may also be transmitted as part of the treatment. This is known as moxibustion; dried mugwort or moxa (*Artemisia vulgaris*), which is tightly packed into a cigarlike stick, is lit and held close to the needle or close to the skin. In many cases, acupuncture treatment involves deep relaxation and can leave you feeling light-headed or sleepy afterward. You may be given dietary advice and offered further treatment depending on your need.

Acupuncture in Labor

Auricular acupuncture involves having a thin needle pushed into the ear or a stud taped over the relevant point. Half-inch needles are inserted into the chosen points and two are attached to an electro-acupuncture machine (Budd 1995). Women are able to control the intensity of the stimulation by themselves, and because the machine is portable they can move around freely.

The points that are stimulated target the relevant area, provide general analgesia throughout the body, and stimulate contractions respectively. After twenty minutes women using it become much calmer and more relaxed.

Although you need an acupuncturist to site them, it is possible to have studs taped in place prior to labor since they only stimulate the points when you press on them.

Acupuncture can also be useful after labor for treating retained placenta and hemorrhoids, increasing the milk supply, and relieving postnatal depression.

• *Fleur Davis* •

The birth of my first child, William, was all right although it could have been better. It was a slow labor and I felt they were eager for me to accept intervention, which I eventually did, although I don't think it was necessary. I would have chosen to have him at home if I had realized how much support was available.

The second time around there was no question of planning for anything but a home birth and I had all my care at home from my midwife, Donna, who got to know us and William well. I felt well looked after and able to call her any time I needed to.

I went into labor three weeks early at a very convenient time; Donna was going to be off duty later and James was due to attend a residential course the following week. The more we thought about it, we realized that the timing was perfect, which made me realize the extent to which the mind can affect labor.

I had felt really ill the day before, hadn't wanted to eat and James said that I was being really unreasonable. I felt funny that night and couldn't sleep. At 1 A.M. I found that I'd had a show and felt very excited, but thought I would not wake anyone. I spent the time cleaning the windows and tidying up, and at two, felt the first distant murmurings of contractions. I started to think about preparing a room for the birth. At six, William got into bed with us and we talked about the baby coming. He wanted it to be a little boy named Thomas, after the Tank Engine.

We called Donna at eight, before she went out on her rounds, and sent my sister to get the TENS machine. Donna came and said that I was 3 cm dilated and having quite strong contractions, and left for a busy day knowing that we could contact her when needed. We walked William to nursery school in the next road and I had two massive contractions on the way that left me clinging to a lamp post wondering whether I would manage to get back.

When we got back, the plumber was fixing the hot water system. When he realized that I was having the baby at home he couldn't get out fast enough and didn't even charge us, saying: "Have a bottle of wine for me!" I put the TENS on far too late and then got on with labor. Staying vertical sped things up and keeping fit during pregnancy with swimming and aerobics helped give me the stamina to cope. Even so, at times I thought that I couldn't do any more although I knew I had to.

Donna came back, found that I was 5 cm and decided to stay. James' sister, who is an acupuncturist, arrived too, and marked me up for points to speed labor; although I was having big contractions I still thought it would be hours. Then I started being sick, which was awful, especially when it coincided with a contraction. Acupuncture helped greatly. Then I had a sudden thought that it might be transition! Donna ruptured my membranes and said I could push if I wanted to. I didn't then, but two contractions later I did.

I found it difficult to get a grip on the floor while I was standing, and Donna suggested that I lean over James' lap on the sofa, which was brilliant. I could feel the head move down to the perineum and felt very clear-headed so that I knew exactly what was going on. The baby's head felt like an enormous wardrobe that I had to get out, and I said "I can't do it", and they all said "You've done it!" and the head was out. It was 12:30.

The room was filled with a beautiful yellow light. James and his sister were crying on the sofa. I didn't turn round at once; I could hear gurgles and knew the baby was all right. Then Donna said: "Your bonus point for the morning is that it is a little girl." I turned around and she was the ugliest thing – all covered in vernix. I just sat and stared at her, all warm, and felt an instant love bond. She pinked up in front of me and at that moment it was just a little girl and me, all alone, and then domesticity returned.

Everyone left us quite suddenly and we were left sitting up in bed in the sunshine wondering what to do with the rest of the afternoon that stretched ahead of us. It was very magical; Madeleine just slipped into our lives. A normal day, but a very special one.

• *Acupressure* •

Acupressure is similar to acupuncture but deep thumb pressure is used instead of needles over the acupuncture points. This has the advantage of making it available to everyone to use, and is preferable for babies and children. It can be useful for use in labor, provided there is someone present who is prepared to press the points. You will know when the right point is reached because it will feel slightly tender and more sensitive than surrounding areas.

Relieving Pain or Speeding Up a Slow Labor
Instructions for a birth partner   Place your thumbs over the acupressure point indicated using the balls of your thumb rather than the tips. Place your weight over them.

- You will find that the correct points are more sensitive than the surrounding areas, and some have slight indentations underneath them.
- As the mother breathes out, build up pressure steadily and evenly over the acupressure points. Maintain the pressure while she holds her breath for three to seven seconds, and then release the pressure as she breathes out. Move on to the next point.
- You can use your elbow gently. This can be useful for large areas such as the buttocks or shoulder muscle.

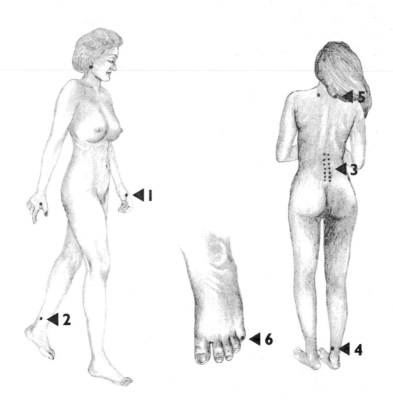

- If you use your fingers, put your index finger on top of your middle finger for more pressure. This is useful if you find that your thumbs are getting tired.

1 On the web of skin between the index finger and the thumb (colon 4). This should only be used for labor. If used before it could cause miscarriage or premature labor.
2 In the groove behind the shin bone, three of the mother's thumb widths above the ankle prominence (spleen 6).
3 Bladder points, either side of the spine, 1½ inches from the groove of the spine, from waist level to her coccyx.
4 The inside of the ankle between the ankle prominence and Achilles tendon (kidney 3). This is good for both postpartum hemorrhage and retained placenta.
5 Points between C7 and the acromium process. Massage all the way along from the point indicated out to the tip of the shoulder. This can be very useful if labor is going slowly.
6 Massage the point at the outer edge of the nail of the little toe at the base of the nail. This may be easiest done with a matchstick.

· TENS ·

The Transcutaneous Electronic Nerve Stimulator (TENS) has become very popular for helping with pain relief in labor because it is under the woman's control, it is drug free, and it can be used at home. It does not have to be administered or approved by anyone else, and it can be stopped instantly if the effect is disliked. A woman using TENS is free to move about and adopt any position, and it can be used in conjunction with breathing and relaxation techniques. It cannot, however, be used in water.

Randomized controlled trials (Carroll 1997) have concluded that TENS has no significant effect on pain in labor, a somewhat surprising finding as the majority of women who find it useful in their labor choose to use it again for subsequent labors. Randomized controlled trials are likely to have given women a real TENS machine or a dummy TENS machine to use once they had reached the hospital in established labor. It is used more satisfactorily when applied at the very start of labor rather than part way through, and availability at home is part of its appeal. A study, which reviewed questionnaires returned to a company that hires out TENS machines, found that of 10,077 respondents, 71 percent reported "excellent" or "good" relief of pain (Johnson M 1997).

The TENS unit, which is also commonly used for chronic pain, works by stimulating the endorphins, the body's natural opiates (see page 30), and also by preventing the message of pain by interfering with the signals sent from the uterus to the brain. Two pairs of electrodes are placed on the back at the spinal levels known as T (thoracic) 10 to L (lumbar) I, and S (sacral) 2 to S4. In the first stage of labor, the sensations that are caused by the contractions of the uterus reach the spinal cord through nerves entering at the level T10–L1, and during the second stage, when pain is felt in the region of the birth canal, the pelvic floor, vagina, and perineum, the messages are sent via nerves entering the spinal cord at the lower level S2 to S4 (where acupuncture points are also located). Electrodes placed over areas of skin that provide sensory input via the spine affect the nerves just under the skin, confusing the message of pain. TENS is thought to partially close a nerve "gateway," so that the full message is not received by the brain.

How to Use TENS Effectively

There are different types of TENS machines. It is important to use an obstetric TENS machine in labor because they have four electrodes. Machines with two are used for other types of pain.

The machine is most effective if put on early; as soon as you are reasonably sure that you are in labor. It can be also be used for back pain or other types of pain associated with late pregnancy. If contractions stop it can easily be removed until they start again.

It is possible to place the self-adhesive electrodes on your back by yourself, but it is easier to have it done by someone else. The electrodes are placed vertically, either side of the spine, about 1½ inches apart with the spine in the middle and with about 3½ inches between the bottom of the upper pair and the top of the lower pair. They are connected via a lead to the TENS machine which can vary in size – the larger ones being the size of a walkman.

The TENS machine is powered by a battery and has two modes: one with intermittent sensation, which stimulates the endorphins, and a continuous mode, which helps prevent the message of pain reaching the brain. When you first put it on you turn up the dial or dials gradually (some have independent controls for the upper and lower pairs of electrodes) until you can feel a sensation that will be tingly or prickly. It is easier to feel in the intermittent mode when you will be aware of a pulsing on your back. Turn the dial carefully to the point where you are aware of the sensation but it is not uncomfortable, then as soon as you feel a contraction, switch the mode to continuous and maintain it until the contraction is over. Then turn it back to intermittent or burst mode.

Within twenty minutes, which is the time it takes to become effective, you will find the sensation on your back has gone. As soon as you cannot feel it any longer, turn it up until you can. If you turn it too high for you at that time it will be too intense, and you will be aware of it. You can either continue to use it like this, alternating between the two modes and increasing the intensity when the sensation fades, or increase the intensity during the contraction and then turn it down afterward. It becomes automatic very quickly and you can use it in whichever way helps you most.

Many women find it a very helpful distraction in the early stages as it gives them something to focus on, and the clicks as they alter the mode of the hand switch lets birth partners know that a contraction has either started or finished.

It is important always to use it at a level where you can feel sensation on your back, and not be tempted to hold it in reserve for later. It works best if you have it up as high as you can manage at the time. Later on, when contractions are getting faster and more intense and there is less break between them, you may find yourself less able to concentrate on manipulating the dial and hand switch. If you reach this point, either someone else can operate it for you – by which time your contractions will probably be obvious to an observer – or you can leave it on the continuous mode until the baby is born.

TENS and Other Pain Relief

You can't use a bath or shower while using TENS, so it is probably best to have one before you put it on. You can take it off, but although the endorphins decline only gradually over several hours, women often find it less effective after a bath, either because labor has progressed or because they are no longer used to handling the contractions with TENS. It is best to turn it off to try a contraction or two without it before getting into water. Women who have had it on right from the start are often unaware of how useful it is proving and find they would prefer to keep it on.

TENS can be used in conjunction with narcotics (such as Demerol) but not with an epidural. If you opt for an epidural while using TENS, it is a good idea to wait until you see the anesthetist before parting with it, or you may have a contraction without either.

TENS may be less helpful in the second stage. It is sometimes described as irritating, but you only need turn it off. It can be useful if you need stitches after your baby is born.

TENS is a method of pain control rather than pain relief. It does not remove pain but can lessen it considerably and is likely to appeal to women who wish to remain in control of their labor, remain mobile, and avoid the use of drugs. It can be particularly useful at home. A TENS machine may be available in the hospital but you will probably need to rent one in order to be able to use it from the start of labor.

• *Self-hypnosis* •

Self-hypnosis – or acquiring a skill that you can use to reduce your awareness of labor pain – provides a safe, drug-free, gentle, and natural form of pain relief.

Hypnotherapists often find it necessary to dispel preconceived ideas about hypnotism exacerbated by television performers who succeed in getting people to act foolishly while apparently in a hypnotic trance. In fact, hypnosis and the ability to put yourself into a hypnotic state are only forms of deep relaxation, similar to meditation or daydreaming. It can only work with your consent and you are neither asleep nor unconscious while you are training yourself in self-hypnosis. The therapist cannot control your mind or your behavior because all hypnosis is self-hypnosis, the therapist merely being the facilitator. It can only be done with your consent when you want it to work. A hypnotherapist will encourage you to relax and focus on a specific area; in this case, labor.

When you enter this state of deep relaxation, you will become more responsive to positive suggestions, cues, or signals given by the therapist. He or she will encourage you to believe in your ability to remain in control and help you to allow your muscles to relax so that your baby's birth can be facilitated in a calm and relaxed way. You will learn how to control levels of tension so that your adrenaline levels do not rise while you are in labor, which can result in a reduced supply of oxygen to the baby (see page 31). When anxiety is eliminated or reduced, the process of birth can be normalized and enhanced, and the body is able to work as intended.

After an initial session, the therapist might give you a tape to take home, so that you and your partner can practice the techniques. The tape will provide positive encouragement and rein-forcement in the belief that you are able to reduce your awareness of pain and relax through painful stimuli while remaining in con-trol. Part of the treatment involves enabling you to visualize the process of birth clearly so that you understand the physiology of birth and see how untensing the muscles can help.

You may be given another tape to work with and will learn tech-niques to put yourself into a state of deep relaxation during labor. Your partner may be taught these as well so that he can help you, if your focus should slip.

Subsequent sessions will enable you to deepen the level of relax-ation that you can achieve, so that by the time the birth comes, you feel fully in control of yourself and confident in your ability to cope.

Benefits for Labor

Anyone can benefit from hypnotherapy preparation for labor, but it is likely to be especially useful for women who are very apprehensive about the prospect, perhaps because of things over-heard in childhood or other prior conditioning, or because of having experienced trauma in a previous birth. It has been estimated that 20 percent of women fear delivery and 6 percent find the fear incapaci-tating. These women may need individual treatment or to find out if there is a qualified hypnotherapist who runs prenatal classes locally.

Women who have used the technique found it helpful, particu-larly because they feel it enabled them to be in control without panic, allowed them freedom to move around, and helped them to feel capable of making decisions that they were happy with subse-quently. Birth partners have also found the training helpful in preparing them by giving them a real sense of confidence and pur-pose in their ability to help and cope during what can be a fright-ening or stressful time.

Some studies suggest that labor is shorter and more satisfying with self-hypnosis. Users may require other pain relief, but do feel very positively about the way their labor went and the fact that they remained in control whatever the circumstances.

• *Sue Hargreaves* •

I conceived as a result of fertility treatment and it was assumed that I would have my baby at the local hospital.

However, I wanted to have a look first and found that I didn't like it. I looked at others but didn't find anywhere that I was happy with. Nowhere seemed conducive to the kind of birth I wanted; I very much wanted to be in control and did not want to hand responsibility over to others.

Eventually I went back to the hospital where I'd had the fertility treatment, which was very open to complementary therapies and offered water birth. It was really lovely there and although it was forty-five minutes' drive from home, I decided to have my baby there and happily changed my prenatal plans. I am only going to have one baby and I wanted it to be right.

However, I do have a history of psychological and health problems: I am an anorexic in recovery, so pregnancy gave me a problem with body image. By about 25 or 26 weeks, I really started panicking about the birth, to such an extent that I told my very understanding doctor that I just couldn't do it any more and that he must get my baby out by cesarean section. I was crying my eyes out, and although he was very reluctant he agreed that he would deliver the baby at 28 weeks because he felt that my psychological symptoms warranted it. He also suggested that I talk to the head of midwifery, and she suggested that I contact a hypnotherapist who ran Birth Without Fear courses. She thought it would be advantageous, even if I did have a cesarean section.

We went to see the hypnotherapist, and I'm so glad we found her because it made such a difference. The work that we did and tapes that I listened to meant that I felt I had control. It was so successful that my doctor could put the cesarean section off each week by suggesting that we leave it for another week, and with both their help I not only managed to get to full term but was overdue.

The birth was brilliant. It started at 6 A.M., although I didn't actually realize; I just had mild period-type pain. I do yoga, and started to practice some of the exercises, but not a lot happened during the course of the morning. By lunchtime I was having intermittent contractions so I stocked up on carbohydrates, because I didn't know what was going to happen, and then sat on the sofa watching television. At 4 o'clock I got up and went to the bathroom, had a sudden pain, and knew that it was labor. Contractions suddenly started coming every four minutes. In the meantime, I listened to the tapes and used visu-

alization techniques. I chose to imagine myself in some gardens in Cornwall and had postcards of them to help my visualization, which was very helpful in the early stages.

We went into the hospital and I had an aromatherapy massage but no other form of pain relief. I particularly did not want Demerol or an epidural because they would mean that I lacked control. The self-hypnosis helped me cope because it made me feel that there was always something that I could do when the pain was severe. Each time it got bad there were other things that I could do, and that gave me the ability to stay on top of the pain. It gave me another piece in my armory and helped me to be focused.

At 9:05 I gave birth to Jonathan. It was a really positive experience. I did feel totally in control and I was so thrilled to feel that I had really done it right. It's given me an awful lot of confidence since and I'm sure that it has made a difference in my attitude to my baby. I was worried that if I had a terrible birth I would have been inclined to blame the baby. As it was I was up and around much quicker than I had expected.

My problems had been heightened, but I think a lot of women fear loss of control. I would recommend self-hypnosis. I don't know what I would have done without it.

Chapter Nine

DRUGS AND PAIN RELIEF

The ideal form of pain relief for labor has not yet been invented. If it had it would have no ill effect on mother or baby either in the short or long term. It would not interfere with the process of labor, would not affect the mother's awareness of what was going on, would not affect her mobility or ability to bear down. It would also be self-administered, giving the mother complete control over it, would be instantly reversible so that she could stop using it whenever she wanted, and its strength could be altered for individual contractions. It would be nonaddictive, and could be used at home (Crafter 1989).

The forms of administered pain relief that are currently available are listed here, with some of their advantages and disadvantages.

• *Demerol* •

Demerol has been used since the 1950s. However, it is falling from favor as research has shown that it is not particularly good at relieving pain, although its sedative effect can mean that it is useful in reducing the tension that women feel when they are not comfortable in their surroundings. It is a synthetic opioid and central nervous system depressant.

Demerol is given by injection. Formerly given in large doses, it is now given in doses of 50 mg, 75 mg, or 100 mg. A dose of 100 mg is equivalent to 10 mg of morphine, but it is shorter-acting. When given intramuscularly, it should take effect within twenty minutes and be most effective after one hour.

Side Effects of Demerol
There are side effects for both mother and baby.

Mother Demerol can cause drowsiness, dizziness, shallow breathing, nausea and vomiting, and slow digestion. It can also cause urine retention. Anti-emetics to prevent nausea and vomiting are often given with Demerol, and antacids may be added to reduce the amount of acid in the stomach. Both the first and second stage have been shown to be longer when Demerol is given (Thomson 1994). In this study, labor was an average of 7.7 hours in the non-Demerol group compared with 11.7 hours in women who had doses of Demerol. (The doses ranged from 75mg to 250mg in total.)

However, many women find most objectionable the sense it can give of loss of control. Women report that they feel "out of it" or disassociated from the birth. They may still feel pain but be less able to respond to it, and some cannot remember what has happened. It can be related to having hallucinations or feeling outside one's body.

Baby Demerol also has well-documented and sometimes long-lasting side effects on the baby. Demerol crosses the placenta easily and babies may be more sensitive to it because of the immaturity of their blood-brain barrier, and because it cannot be metabolised in their liver before birth.

The effect of Demerol is most marked when given two to three hours before birth, when it depresses the rate of respiration (breathing difficulties). Babies are likely to have lower Apgar scores at birth and be sleepy and unresponsive for a few days after birth. This can mean that they show less interest in feeding, making breast-feeding harder to establish.

One study (Belsey 1981) found that differences between babies who had received high levels of Demerol during birth continued to show effects of the drugs for six weeks afterward: they were more likely to cry during tests, to be less settled and less able to quiet themselves. The effects of Demerol were most noticeable when the babies were seven days old, particularly in those who had received higher doses. Another study (Jacobson 1990) found that children of women who had used both Demerol and morphine barbiturates in labor were more likely to become addicted to opiates as an adult than those whose mothers had not taken drugs which crossed the placenta.

It is possible to reverse the adverse effects of Demerol in a baby by giving it an injection of naloxone (Narcan) intramuscularly immediately after birth. However, the effect lasts for up to forty-eight hours whereas the effects from Demerol last longer (Wiener 1977), but babies who have been given the antidote are more likely to feed and so excrete the drug more rapidly.

It is less well known that Narcan can be given to a laboring women if she has been given Demerol and dislikes its effect.

Effectiveness of Demerol

In short, Demerol is not very effective at relieving pain, although it can relax muscles that may be tense as a result of labor or the situation in which labor is taking place. In a study of 663 women (Holdcroft 1974), 75 percent said they had little or no pain relief from Demerol. You may be offered it readily, but it has significant disadvantages both to you and your baby. Good support is said to be at least as effective as Demerol.

• *Joan Jones* •

I found what really helped with labor pain was experience. I had my first child seventeen years ago and a lot of time was spent at prenatal classes practicing breathing levels. I absorbed the idea that if I breathed perfectly it wouldn't hurt. (Whether this was the idea the teacher was trying to put over I don't know.) I was very frightened of labor and found the session on pain relief terrifying as I was sure that I didn't like any of the options.

When labor started I was appalled to discover that what I thought was excruciating pain was a "weak contraction", and what I was reacting to with desperate breathing was "only the baby moving". I was completely panicked and Demerol didn't help, only made me drunk and sick. Second stage, however, was fine; I really enjoyed it except that I had a large tear.

The second labor, fifteen years ago, was induced with prostaglandin gel and artificial rupture of the membranes got it going. I was coping well with the contractions but didn't like the continuous ache in my cervix. (Was this caused by the gel or the "sweep"?) I was offered Demerol and was persuaded by my partner to take it and spent the rest of the labor completely "out of it". I then had a postpartum hemorrhage and a blood transfusion.

The third baby, born thirteen years ago, was a posterior presentation again, as the first had been. This labor started at night; we went to the same hospital, just at the right time and I coped easily with contractions. I knew how they were going to feel, the midwife was great and took no notice when I groaned a bit. By this time, NO DEMEROL was written on my notes in large red letters. I was so pleased with myself that when Alan

decided to come out "sunny side up" (persistent occipito-poste-
rior or POP), and I discovered that second stage was hurting,
I was disgusted. I had never had a painful second stage before
and it wasn't fair! But it didn't last long and I coped fine.

The fourth and last labor (she's now eleven) was induced
again. I asked for this myself (heresy I know) because my
mother-in-law couldn't stay much longer and I'd been having
contractions for an hour every morning for the last week. Like
the second labor, it was quick. After the insertion of the gel,
contractions set in, ARM helped and Lucy appeared at 11:10
A.M. This was the one I really enjoyed. I really felt I knew what
I was doing and it didn't seem to hurt.

During this labor I had a very mysterious experience.
Because labor was going so fast I declined to move about and
curled up on my side on the bed. It seemed to me that "I" was
a very small person in the middle of "my body," which was a
huge cavernous room. The contractions were like gales of roar-
ing wind blowing through, but I felt quite safe curled up there
in the middle of this vast space. And I don't remember pain at
all, though I did decide to experiment with giving birth kneel-
ing and found the pressure of the head very uncomfortable.

• *Amarit Kahn* •

I went into labor at 10 o'clock at night and went to the hospi-
tal at 3 A.M. because I was having really severe pains. When I
got there they found that I was a few centimetres dilated and
everything was progressing nicely and painfully. I used the
TENS machine to help distract me from the pain.

By nine that morning, they were pleased with my progress
and told us that the baby would be born by about lunchtime, so
we called our family to let them know. Then the staff offered
me Demerol to help me with the last bit. It was given to me as
a patient controlled outfit so that I just had to press a button
to get a bit more of the drug. It seemed to knock me out imme-
diately; my husband said that I was jabbering away and that
my eyes were rolling around. I felt as if I was floating all over
the place. I was drifting in and out of consciousness, and came
to to find the midwife shouting at me to get me to come round.
The labor had stopped progressing as soon as I'd had it, and

*after five hours of no further progress they gave me Pitocin to
get it going again. He was finally born at 5:30 that evening,
but I felt I had lost five or six hours in a daze.*

*Then I tore, and it took two hours to stitch me up with my
legs in stirrups all the time. I wasn't able to see or feed my baby
and I feel robbed by that more than anything. He was very
sleepy all that night, but fine the following morning, so it had
affected me more than him – but I really wish that I hadn't had it.*

· *Epidural* ·

An epidural is an injection of anesthetic into the epidural space
around your spinal cord, close to the nerves that convey the message of labor pain to the brain. When it works well it can reduce all
the pain of labor while leaving you some sensation in your legs.
Recent developments mean that it is possible to give low doses of
anesthetic so that you are still able to walk around while receiving
the benefit of pain relief. This is known as the mobile epidural.

The epidural has to be inserted with care by a skilled anesthesiologist. It can be difficult to remain still while it is administered but
should be effective within twenty minutes. It provides the most
complete form of pain relief but is also the most invasive and can
only be given in a hospital setting. Although many women are very
satisfied with an epidural there can be some disadvantages, both
physical and emotional.

Because an epidural has to be given by an anesthesiologist,
there may be a delay between deciding to have one and actually
receiving it.

In order to have an epidural you have to sit on the edge of the
bed sitting forward or lying in a fetal position which can be hard to
maintain during a contraction. Your back will be cleaned and then
you will be given a local anesthetic before a wide bore needle is
carefully inserted into your spine in the lumbar region. Once it is in
place in the epidural space, a fine polyethylene tube is threaded in
through the needle, which is then removed and the tube is taped in
place up your back. A cap is fitted to the end of the tube to seal it.
A small test dose will be given first and then if all is well the drug
(bupivacaine) is given. As it goes in you may feel a cold trickle
down your back, and then after about twenty minutes your feet will
become warm and the pain of contractions will fade. Some women
react with trembling, the epidural shakes. You may have to be

turned from side to side to ensure that the drug is evenly distributed. Although most epidurals are effective, some do not work at all and some leave some residual, patchy pain so that it might work on one side but not the other. In studies, 6 to 8 percent of women found them to be of little or no use.

Mobile Epidural

In many maternity units, the mobile epidural is available, in which lower doses of drugs are used, but are topped off more frequently. The advantages include the fact that you do not lose sensation in your legs so that you are able to walk around with it in place. However, studies have shown no difference in the rate of spontaneous vaginal delivery between those with a mobile epidural and those with the standard epidural or when mobility is not possible. In first-time mothers the rate was 43 percent in both groups, but there was an increase from 1 percent to 2 percent in women who had a dural puncture headache (see page 124), and lowered blood pressure rates increased from 9 percent to 14 percent.

Side Effects of Epidurals

There are also some side effects (which may be less severe as lower doses of drugs are used) but they include the fact that Pitocin is used three times as much on women with an epidural as those without, and the length of the second stage of labor is significantly increased. There is also a threefold increase in the number of instrumental deliveries, that is, forceps or vacuum extraction. This is because the urge to push is not felt, so that pushing has to be done consciously. It is possible to wait for the baby's head to be visible before starting pushing, and/or for the epidural to be allowed to wear off although this can result in the return of pain. If pushing is started while the head is still high, rotational forceps are more likely to be needed.

The cesarean-section rate caused by the baby becoming stuck is doubled with an epidural. It can also be responsible for removing sensation from the bladder so that a catheter has to be inserted.

An epidural can be responsible for a fall in blood pressure, which may be useful if your blood pressure is raised, but up to 2 percent of women require ephedrine to treat it. Epidurals can raise a woman's temperature – which may have an effect in raising the baby's heartbeat. It can also mean that the baby may be tested for infection after birth.

In extremely rare cases, some women may be permanently damaged by an epidural, with potentially life-threatening complications of labor occurring in one in 4,000 women in labor. Sensory loss and weakness occur afterward in four to eighteen per 10,000 women, most improving within three months. Many women suspect that they have long-term back pain after an epidural, although there is no clear evidence of a link. In the short term there is a 1 percent risk of the needle accidentally puncturing the dura, which can result in a headache, which may be very severe and require nursing flat on your back for up to ten days.

Satisfaction with Labor

Epidurals are popular because they take away the pain and make labor easier not only for the mother, but also her caregivers who often find looking after someone who is in a lot of pain is both taxing and emotionally draining. Many women are delighted with them but, perhaps surprisingly, effective pain relief does not necessarily result in a satisfactory birth experience. Prenatal teachers often hear birth after epidural described as being rather flat and anticlimatic because there is no sense of achievement of mastery over the pain.

Barbara Morgan, anesthesiologist at Queen Charlotte's Maternity Hospital in London, surveyed 1,000 women who had given birth there and found that those who were least satisfied with their birth experience were those who had had epidurals. They felt the same a year after their babies' births, and there was a correlation behind long labor, subsequent forceps delivery, and dissatisfaction. There is no way of knowing whether labor would have been long or forceps unnecessary without the epidural but it was clear that many felt that they were deprived of the experience of giving birth.

Those survey results have caused maternity services to reevaluate the rate of pain relief in labor, because for a long time it was assumed that removal of pain would result in total satisfaction, as was suggested by the enthusiasm with which the early forms of pain relief – such as chloroform – were greeted. Although it is sometimes believed that an epidural means that the baby does not receive any of the drug, this is not the case.

Bupivacaine does cross the placenta and can affect babies and their behavior for up to six weeks; they are likely to cry more easily, be less alert, and have poorer visual skills. They are more likely to be irritable on the third day after birth and are less able to quiet themselves. On the other hand, muscle tone seems to be improved although motor organization is impaired. The more bupivacaine that a woman is given the greater the effect on the baby (Rosenblatt 1981).

Epidurals can be a valuable form of pain relief, particularly in abnormal labors, which can be unusually painful. However, they do have the most associated side effects, and their use can cause later regrets. If you want to avoid one, make sure that maternity staff are aware of the fact so that they can help you to manage without it.

• *Sue Weston* •

I really wanted my baby to be on time, so when I went into labor two days before I was due I thought it might be wishful thinking. I'd had what felt like bad period pains for the previous couple of days and contractions started on Wednesday morning just before I was due to meet the girls from my prenatal class for coffee. They were feeling sorry for me because they had all had their babies, so they were very excited to think it might be happening. They helped me to put my TENS machine on correctly and I went home and sat around for a while. I found sitting propped up with cushions most helpful

Eventually, I called the hospital to warn that I might be coming in, and my husband came home. The hospital said "Don't leave it too late, but if you feel all right, have something to eat and stay at home a bit longer."

My bag had been packed since 32 weeks but Richard had to sort out the rugby team for Saturday, so he was doing that in between timing contractions and making us sandwiches. The contractions felt like a weird low-down squeeze-cum-period pain; later they felt like bands of elastic tightening. At 4 P.M. we left in order to avoid the rush hour.

It was lovely and quiet when we got there and we were admitted straight into the delivery room. The TENS machine worked until 6 P.M. I definitely had not wanted an epidural, but by 7 P.M. I was asking for one. The anesthesiologist was with us in fifteen minutes although the drug wasn't in until 8.

I was offered either a full or a mobile epidural, but by then I was happy to have whatever they thought was best. They suggested the mobile and I sat up bent over cushions while it was inserted. We were both very worried about something going wrong, so I remained very still while it was done although it was extremely difficult. It started to work quite quickly. The pain in my ribs where I had felt the baby's feet for weeks went quickly, although I was left with an area around the pubic bone where it was not effective, which was very painful, especially when I thought it would be the answer to all my problems.

Then my waters suddenly went, increasing the pain and giving me terrible shakes. They were stained with green meconium, which worried me because I thought the baby might be in distress and I might need a cesarean. Fortunately, the baby's heartbeat was all right, and by turning me from side to side the epidural was made to work fully and I stopped shaking. The drug was topped off every forty-five minutes or so, and I progressed from 3 to 7 cm quite quickly. At this point – 10:45 P.M. – the vice-captain called to finalize a few details about Saturday's match!

By midnight they said I could push, although I was worried about bad pain and shaking returning. The drug was topped off and I started pushing at 3 A.M. I couldn't feel what to do at first, but eventually I managed it and contractions speeded up. It was really hard work – like sprint training without a break – for an hour and a half. It wasn't painful but it felt like one step forward and two backward, although they said I was doing well. I have good lung capacity, being used to playing rugby and running, and managed four pushes with every contraction. I thought that they were lying, but eventually I could feel intense pressure on my perineum and realized the head wasn't going back. Once they said they could see the head I knew I could do it.

They told me to start panting, which I could manage because the urge to push was not too strong. Once the head was out the baby shot out. Richard shouted "Its a boy!" and was more emotional than me. I felt completely exhausted and shell-shocked and relieved that it was all over. I was almost more pleased that I only needed two stitches.

I had originally worried that I would let myself down by having an epidural because I had been convinced that I would manage without. In the end, I didn't feel guilty because it took away the pain, and I felt that the mobile was the in-between option.

Chapter Ten

EPISIOTOMIES AND TEARS

An episiotomy is a cut made by a midwife or doctor into your perineum in order to enlarge the outlet for the baby. It is done by injecting local anesthetic into the perineum and then cutting it with very sharp scissors. In an emergency there may not be time to give the anesthetic, but the pressure of the baby's head has a numbing effect so that you probably would not feel the cut.

An episiotomy may be necessary if the baby is distressed and needs to be delivered rapidly; if your tissues are so rigid that they are holding the baby in; or perhaps if it looks as though you are going to tear badly, although an episiotomy does not necessarily prevent tearing. An episiotomy is usually made for a forceps delivery, and may be made when the baby is premature or when its bottom or shoulder is the presenting part.

Episiotomies are often regarded with alarm by women who feel very apprehensive at the thought of having a cut in such a sensitive area. Unfortunately their fears can be justified because they can cause considerable pain after the birth, hinder breast-feeding, and sometimes make the days and even weeks afterward miserable.

You can take steps to prevent episiotomy or tearing by massaging your perineum beforehand (see pages 128–129) but to some extent your best guard against an episiotomy is a midwife or doctor who takes pride in helping women to give birth with an intact perineum. They will make sure that you do not push too vigorously or for too long and that you do not consciously push until your baby's head is on your perineum, and they will help you to breathe the baby out gently through relaxed perineal muscles.

It is useful to discuss episiotomy while you are in labor even though you may have it on your birth plan. Make sure that your midwife knows what you would prefer; you may prefer a tear to a cut if a laceration cannot be avoided. There is some evidence that tearing along the line of least resistance is more satisfactory, in terms of healing and pain, than an episiotomy. A straight cut is easier to stitch but a tear can be fitted together like a jigsaw and may feel a bit more comfortable. If a tear does occur you know that it has been necessary.

Many midwives can suture – and you may prefer to have your midwife put in any stitches that are needed. Some midwives feel that all but the most severe tears heal best unsutured, provided the mother rests in bed during the process. Medical students first learn to suture on a torn or cut perineum; you can say if you would prefer to have it done by a senior doctor. It should be done very soon after the birth and involves you lying on your back with your legs supported by stirrups, at the end of the delivery bed.

Your perineum is injected with local anaesthetic and the wound stitched with sutures that are designed to be absorbed by your skin as it heals. It can take up to an hour, depending on the degree of repair.

The stitches may be comfortable to start with but can become very painful as they start to heal and you feel the effects of bruising. If you have had a large episiotomy you may find walking and sitting miserable and it can make trying to feed your baby very uncomfortable. It has been shown that pain from stitches reduces the number of women breast-feeding (Rajan 1994). The pain can be underestimated by midwifery staff – make sure that they know how you are feeling and if you need extra help with breast-feeding. They will be able to find ways of making sitting more comfortable.

You can try and make a cut or tear unnecessary by practicing perineal massage in the last few weeks of pregnancy. You can start at around 30 weeks but it is still worth doing even if you are nearer to the end of pregnancy. This has been shown to be beneficial (Shipman 1997) in reducing tears or episiotomies and instrumental deliveries, with increasing benefit for those over the age of thirty.

• *Perineal Massage* •

The best time to do perineal massage is following a warm bath when your tissues are softer. Using an oil – such as almond, comfrey, olive, vitamin E, or wheatgerm – lubricate your fingers, then very gently insert two fingers into your vagina and gradually increase the space between them so that the skin becomes stretched – a bit like pulling out the corners of your mouth. You will find that as time goes by you will be able to accommodate more of your fingers as your skin becomes more supple. Hook your thumbs into your vagina and pull the perineum outward, massaging the skin with the oil in a U-shape while concentrating particularly on any area of tenderness or previous scar tissue. You will find that the whole area softens as your body prepares to give birth, but massaging daily, for 15 minutes or more, can make a real difference to your perineum.

· *Healing Cuts and Tears* ·

There are a number of remedies to help with the healing of cuts or tears. It is a good idea to have them ready before the birth, as you will not feel like organizing it afterward. If you find they are not needed, you should nevertheless consider it money well spent.

Take an Arnica 200 tablet (see pages 99, 102–103) when you are in the second stage of labor – you will need someone to remind you – and one just after the birth. Thereafter, take one whenever you feel bruised or sore; the symptoms should improve. If they return take another, so that they are not taken at set intervals but in response to your need. You should not have anything to eat and drink for about twenty minutes before and after taking the tablet. Some women find that applying hot, wet washcloths or compresses to the perineum, just before the head crowns, helps their tissues to stretch.

Practical Suggestions for Healing Perineal Damage
- Keep stitches as clean as possible.
- Ask your midwife if there is anything available to help. Ultrasound treatment is sometimes available in the hospital. If the pain relief you are receiving is not adequate tell your midwife or doctor. The severity of pain is often underestimated.
- If you find it soothing you can apply icepacks: crushed ice in bags, frozen peas, water frozen in a rubber glove so a finger can be inserted into the vagina.
- A handful of salt in the bath can act as an antiseptic.
- Sit in bowls of hot and cold water alternately.
- Add 6 drops of a 50:50 mix of essential oils of lavender and cypress to a shallow bath or wash bowl and sit in it as long as needed.
- To soothe and heal use a tincture of calendula and/or hypericum (St John's Wort) diluted in water 1:10 as a perineal wash.
- You can make a paste with slippery elm bark powder and comfrey root powder mixed with olive oil, vitamin E oil, and water. Spread it on to muslin and hold it in place with a pad, and change

it every time you go to the bathroom.
- Once the wound has healed you can massage the area gently with calendula cream, vitamin E, or comfrey oils to assist further healing and reduce the amount of scar tissue.

Homeopathic Remedies
- Bellis Perennis 200 for tears. Take one dose; it works deeper than Arnica.
- Staphisagria 30. Take doses after an episiotomy, particularly if you feel resentful about having had it done.
- Pyrogen 30. Take this for as long as needed if your perineum was cut or tore, and is failing to heal.

Herbal Bath Use a combination of shepherd's purse, comfrey, and uva ursi. A handful each of the dried herbs should be added to a large pan of water, together with a cup of sea salt and three heads of peeled and pricked cloves of garlic. Bring to the boil and simmer for just over half an hour. Strain and mash the juice in a muslin cloth and add the mixture to a shallow bath. Sit in it until the pain is relieved. You may add a few drops of the fluid extract of the herbs to the boiled and cooled salt and garlic if it is easier. This recipe should be used for several days following the birth.

Aftereffects The stitches should dissolve naturally but your midwife can snip them after a few days if they continue to cause trouble. They can often feel worse while the skin tightens and itches as it heals.

It is important to ask your midwife or doctor if you have any concerns about your perineal wound. Don't suffer in silence if you think there is something wrong; ask to be referred to a gynecologist if it is still causing trouble by six weeks.

If you find sex difficult because there is a lack of lubrication you can use KY Jelly, and you may need practice and patience before you are back to normal.

Chapter Eleven

CESAREAN SECTION

Cesarean section has been around for a long time. Its name is derived from the Latin verb, *caedere* – to cut. The operation was known in Roman times, but it was not until 1882, when chloroform became available to dull the pain, that women with deformed pelvises could be delivered this way. By 1958 only 2.7 percent of babies were born this way. By 1970 the rates in the U.S. and England were around 5 percent but there has since been a dramatic escalation so that rates of 25 percent are the norm in the U.S. The World Health Organization's view (WHO 1985) is that no country should have a rate of more than 10 percent.

These rates are horribly high and cannot be a reflection of a massive increase in birth complications. Clearly, something is wrong if fewer than three out of four women are deemed capable of giving birth outside an operating room.

• *Essential cesareans* •

Some women and their babies clearly fall into the category where cesarean section is essential to save life. These include:

- Cord prolapse: when the cord comes down in front of the baby.
- Placenta previa: the placenta blocks the cervix at the time of delivery (although this should be checked just before a cesarean section is performed as it is possible for the diagnosis to alter as the uterus grows).
- Placental abruption: when the placenta peels away from the wall of the uterus before the baby is born.
- Preeclampsia, also known as toxemia: a syndrome that includes very high blood pressure, protein in the urine, and sometimes fluid retention. If untreated, it can result in a decrease in the supply of oxygen to the baby and convulsions in the mother. It is potentially fatal.
- Transverse lie: if the baby lies across the uterus instead of vertically, and cannot be persuaded to alter its position, it has to be delivered by cesarean section.

- Contracted pelvis: cesarean may be necessary if your pelvis has been damaged in an injury such as a car accident, or it has been deformed by disease such as rickets or osteomalacia.
- Interuterine Growth Retardation: cesareans are done for babies that are very small because they have not grown properly and may find the stress of labor too much. However, estimates of fetal size done by ultrasound can be quite inaccurate.
- Medical conditions of the baby: there are some rare conditions in babies that mean that they will find it hard to survive birth or it will be impossible for them to pass through the birth canal; for example heart conditions, hydrocephalus, or other conditions where the baby is not formed normally.

Making a Choice

If a cesarean section is suggested to you it will not be presented as a choice. You therefore have to make up your own mind, which can be very difficult. If you have time, you will need information (see support groups listed on page 149) and can seek a second opinion, either from another obstetrician within the unit or elsewhere, via your primary care physician. Ask your midwife for her advice. Ask for your unit's cesarean section rate. If it is high, you may be better off at a unit where it is lower.

Here is a list of conditions which are sometimes treated by cesarean section: breech presentation; existing medical condition; failure to progress; multiple birth; herpes; HIV-positive mother; premature labor; unstable lie; disability; cephalopelvic disproportion (that is, baby's head too big for mother's pelvis); fibroids; previous stillbirth or miscarriage; previous cesarean.

• *The Operation* •

During the week before you will be given a blood test to check your hemoglobin levels. Your obstetrician will explain the operation to you and ask you to sign a consent form. You will be given two tablets to take before the operation to reduce the acidity in your stomach while you are being operated on. This is to reduce the risk of aspirating the contents of your stomach (see page 73).

On the day of the operation you should have a bath or shower, remove any makeup, nail polish or jewelery: the anesthesiologist needs to be able to see the true color of your lips and nails.

Most planned cesareans are carried out under spinal or

epidural anesthesia because of the advantages that it has for you and your baby physically, and because you will be awake and able to see your baby the minute he or she is born. A general anesthetic may be used in an emergency, when the baby shows signs of acute distress, and is necessary if spinal or epidural anesthesia is not possible for any reason. However it has the disadvantage that it can make you drowsy and confused for several days afterward; you are not aware of the baby's birth; you can have a sore throat and congested chest as a result of the way the anesthetic is given; and the baby may be floppy or have breathing difficulties. Afterward, breast-feeding can be harder to establish and it is rare for hospitals to allow partners to be present when a woman is given a general anesthetic.

You will have various routine tests done and a blood sample taken for cross matching, and your pubic hair will be shaved around the bikini line. You will then be given a clean gown to wear and elasticized stockings to put on which help to reduce the risk of a clot developing afterward. Your partner will be given surgical scrubs to put on and you will both be taken to the operating room. A drip will be put in the back of your hand via a needle which is strapped to the back of it, and then you will be given the epidural (see page 122). It will take up to thirty minutes to take effect.

Once it is working you will have a catheter inserted into your bladder to keep it empty during surgery. Just before the operation starts, you will be given a drink of sodium citrate to further reduce the acidity of your stomach.

A screen will be placed between you and your abdomen, and once the surgeon is confident that you cannot feel any pain, he or she will begin. You will feel the cut like someone drawing a pencil across your skin at the bikini line, and you may feel a sensation of rummaging as the baby is taken out of you. Within a few minutes, he or she will be held up for you to see, and then be dried and examined quickly before being given to you to hold and admire. While you are cuddling your baby, the placenta will be removed, and you will be given Pitocin.

After that, your baby will be weighed, measured, bathed, and dressed warmly. During this time your incision will be stitched, which takes about thirty minutes. When it is complete you can breast-feed your baby. You and your partner and your baby will be moved to a nearby delivery room for half an hour or more for observation to make sure that you are not suffering from any complications. If all is well you will then be taken to the maternity ward.

• *After the Operation* •

You will be given some kind of pain-reliever at the end of the operation and may also be given antibiotics via drip to reduce the risk of infection. The anesthetic effect wears off after a few hours and you will be given further pain relief, either through a drip, as injections, more suppositories, or as a liquid or tablets. TENS (see page 111) can be useful in relieving pain in the area of the wound, when electrodes are placed either side of it.

You will be in pain after the operation and may be surprised to find how difficult it is just to move. Because your stomach muscles have been cut it can be hard to turn over or sit up, and you will need help to pick up and hold your baby and with breast-feeding. Although women often recover surprisingly quickly, particularly after a planned cesarean, it is normal to find things a struggle. Someone else will change your baby and help will be available until you can manage by yourself. Do not hesitate to ask for help when you need it.

Although pain relief after cesarean section is usually freely available – perhaps more so than for equally painful perineal stitches – you should ask for it if you feel you need it, and not compare your recovery with that of other cesarean-birth women.

Getting in and out of bed can be very difficult after the operation and it can be very hard to stand up straight and walk. It may demand all your strength just to get a short distance down the corridor and you may feel that other people fail to understand your problems. Maternity staff are used to dealing with these problems and can, if asked, supply aids to help you, including extra pillows, a stool by the side of your bed, and an adjustable height crib for the baby so that it is easier for you to get him or her out by yourself.

You will be encouraged to become mobile quickly to reduce the risk of developing deep vein thrombosis (clots) which can be a serious complication, more common after cesareans. You can usually expect to be drinking normally, eating a light diet, and walking to the lavatory with help when needed by the time your baby is 24 hours old. Your intravenous drips and catheter will be removed as soon as possible and you can have a shower.

Because cesareans are so common these days you may find that people consider that you have got away lightly because you have not been through labor, be envious because you have avoided labor pain, or just regard it as no big deal. Because it is a way of giving birth and the baby can be the focus of attention, there may be very little recognition that you have had a major abdominal operation as well as a baby, and consequently require physical and emotional support. It is quite interesting to compare the after-care and expectations of what women can do following hysterectomy with those who have had cesareans.

It is important that your family realizes what you can and can't do. You should have help at home at least for the first few days, or longer if you need it, or if you have been discharged when your baby is only days old.

Although many women are quite content with the way their baby has been delivered, others may feel great resentment, particularly if they had been working toward a natural birth or did not feel part of the decision to operate. It is very important to discuss the reasons for and your feelings about the birth with the people who were concerned with it – doctors or midwives – so that you know exactly why it was done and can be sure it was necessary. You can also ask whether they think it would be needed in another pregnancy and what their policy is on vaginal birth following cesarean. This opportunity for discussion, which should be offered to you while you are still in hospital, can be requested at any time afterward and can be a very important part of your recovery.

The amount of pain that you feel will gradually diminish although it may take several months so that you may reach a point where you forget that it is not normal. It is important to pace yourself and make sure that you eat well after a cesarean. Don't be afraid to ask for help with household tasks and food preparation; your priorities should be looking after yourself and your baby. If you are breast-feeding, ask for any help that you need from a midwife, breast-feeding counselor, or health visitor and appreciate that it may be more difficult to start with. It is best to be realistic about what you can achieve and not risk getting overexhausted.

Chapter Twelve

POSTPARTUM PAIN

When you visualize yourself sitting up in bed holding your new baby, you do not usually image yourself being in acute discomfort as well. However, this will probably be the case – not surprisingly when you consider the changes that your body has been through. The effect of giving birth, the huge change in hormone levels, and the emotional weight of the experience, can all contribute to early motherhood as being a difficult and stressful time, as well as a time of great joy– although one study found that only 31 percent of women described themselves pleased with their new baby while other reactions varied from mixed to disgusted.

In the later stages of pregnancy women are often eager to have the baby soon because they find life so uncomfortable, imagining that once the baby is born they will feel as they did before they became pregnant. Unfortunately, in reality it can seem as if you have just exchanged one set of discomforts for another. Moreover, the labor is such a big experience that you may find it hard to remember how uncomfortable you may have been before it started. There is also the other consideration that your baby – hitherto quiet and fed automatically – now needs caring for at the same time as you are recovering from the birth.

You are likely to feel as if you are leaking from every orifice. Temperatures need to be quite high for the baby's sake (61 to 68°F), and this means that you will sweat off much of the extra 3½ pints of fluid of late pregnancy, as well as urinating copious amounts. Blood loss from the vagina, known as lochia, which comes from the place where the placenta was attached to your uterus – can be heavy with large clots, and after a couple of days you will find that milk leaks readily from your breasts, soaking breast pads. If you have stitches, either in the perineum or across your abdomen they can be very painful, and the days when your breasts are engorged as the milk come in can be very trying. You may also be suffering from after-pains, especially if it is not your first baby.

Many women find it impossible to sleep after the birth, no matter how much sleep they have lost during labor. This is particularly likely if endorphin levels have not been reduced by an epidural. They may feel a terrific high to start with, which wears off after a couple of days, leading to the third-day baby blues. At the same time, the baby is likely to become less sleepy and wake up more frequently for feeding, noticeably at night.

If mothering is new to you, you will also have an overwhelming feeling of responsibility and concern for the well-being of your baby, which can make it much harder to relax and let go when you do get the opportunity to sleep.

Looking After the Mother

Added to these problems is the possibility that you may be suffering from backache and sore nipples, be finding feeding difficult to establish, and that the baby may cry on and off for a lot longer than you want. It is no wonder that you may not be feeling wonderful. Mothers at this stage need mothering themselves, and the fortunate ones are looked after by their families.

Only 20 years ago, women having a first baby were expected to stay in the hospital for several days afterward and had to get written permission from their doctor if they wanted to leave any earlier. Since then, pregnancy has lost a lot of its mystique and women expect and are expected to have little time off before the birth and to leave the hospital shortly afterward. The current belief that pregnancy does not hamper you in any way, and the lack of tolerance of a period of recovery or provision of any special assistance for new mothers, goes against centuries of tradition, and can contribute to women's feelings of inadequacy after the birth.

The period of support that women were traditionally accorded – a month or more, whether it was actually possible to observe it or not – shows an understanding of the complexity of adaptation to new motherhood and a recognition of the amount of time that caring for a new baby takes. Although few women would care to consider themselves polluted, let alone lie unwashed on a straw mattress for three weeks, very many would appreciate a greater understanding of their needs and practical assistance with their new baby in its early days. Although early ambulation is encouraged to prevent the formation of potentially fatal thromboses (of which descriptions in history are interestingly rare), it seems as though the baby has been thrown out with the bath water, as brief stays in hospital are equated in the public mind with little or no need for rest at home subsequently.

If you find that the sum total of having given birth together with caring for and sustaining a new life is making you feel awful, accept any help that is offered. Although you probably won't think so, other people can look after the baby for a short while. And, if the baby is depending on you for all its food, it needs you at your best, fittest, and most relaxed. There is a direct link between how much you eat, the amount of energy that you expend, and the supply of milk available for the baby. Your baby depends on you so it is important to rest, eat well, and rest again. Let other people look after the household – it is only a very short time – about six weeks before your body sorts itself out, the baby's feeding patterns are recognizable, and motherhood becomes a pleasure. By the time your baby is smiling you will feel far better.

If you find life difficult say so – do not suffer in silence, or imagine that every other new mother is coping. Ask for help; most people feel very benign towards new babies and are glad to give it.

• *Postpartum Hemorrhage* •

Blood loss at birth is normal, but the amount is calculated; more than 500 ml is considered to constitute a postpartum hemorrhage (PPH). To lose blood like that can be a terrifying experience – it can either be in a gush or persistent trickle – and your midwife will treat it by giving you an injection that will cause the uterus to contract within forty seconds and reduce the bleeding. If you lose a lot of blood you will need a blood transfusion.

It is worth taking iron supplements after a PPH, even if they are not suggested, because they can make a lot of difference to the way you feel. Anemia can add to the exhaustion of early motherhood. You can buy iron in capsule form from the drugstore, or may prefer a preparation in which the iron is supplied by a mixture of herbs.

Occasionally you may have a secondary PPH, in the weeks after the baby is born. If you experience a sudden heavy loss of blood, contact a midwife immediately or call for an ambulance.

• *Lochia* •

This is the blood loss that is normal following birth, whether vaginally or by cesarean section. It can be dauntingly heavy to start with and may contain large clots. You will need very absorbent pads to cope with it. Tampons are not recommended because of the risk of increasing infection in what is effectively an open wound in your uterus. Suitable pads are sold as maternity pads. You will probably need several packages as you will need to change one every time you go to the bathroom.

Contact your midwife if at any time you feel that you are bleeding excessively (see PPH). You can expect bleeding to be brighter and heavier as you become more active but it gradually changes in color from red to red-brown and then to almost colorless as the area to which the placenta was attached heals. It can take four to six weeks to stop altogether. If the lochia becomes foul-smelling, or you have other signs of infection such as a raised temperature, feel as if you have flu, or have headaches or pain in the area of your uterus, contact your doctor or midwife right away. Infections of this kind need to be treated with antibiotics immediately.

• *Afterpains* •

The uterus continues to contract in the days after birth until it is eventually the same size as it was before you were pregnant. Although you are less likely to be aware of it following a first baby, the contractions of the uterus when it shrinks can be as painful as those of labor and are most noticeable when you breast-feed because the release of oxytocin stimulates the contractions. They tend to get stronger in intensity after each pregnancy, so they may be severe. Taking Arnica 200 (see pages 98–102) seems to make a difference, both in the amount of pain and the quantity of blood lost after a birth, and is well worth a try. If you do not have it, you may want to take acetaminophen to see you through the early days.

• *Bowels* •

If you have had stitches, either abdominal or perineal, the first bowel movement after giving birth can be an alarming prospect. Although your stitches will not give way, you can easily feel that they might and the extra pressure increases the pain.

It is quite common to be constipated for a few days after giving birth anyway because you are likely to have had diarrhea before labor started, probably not eaten a lot of fiber-containing food during labor, and the fluid that you lose as urine and sweat can reduce the bulk of the stool, making it harder. However, it cannot be delayed forever and there are steps that you can take to make it easier. If you are really bothered, take two acetaminophen tablets at least half an hour beforehand. Try to be as relaxed as possible (make sure that someone else is looking after your baby) and use the breathing technique that helped in labor.

You may find that it helps to lubricate the area in and just outside the anus with petroleum jelly and to hold a clean pad firmly over the stitch line. It can be easier if you lean to one side taking the pressure off one buttock. Alternatively, you can try squatting with one or both feet on or beside the lavatory seat; at home you can put an upturned bucket on either side, or use a potty.

With an abdominal wound, when your concern is using pressure on the abdominal muscles to bear down, it can help to lean forward with your hand firmly over the stitches.

If these tactics do not work – and it may take several attempts – there are other measures. Your midwife will be able to supply laxative suppositories or you can buy them at the drugstore. She can give you an enema if you are desperate. It is best not to take laxatives orally as they can be excreted in breast milk, although there are products which increase the bulk of the stool by adding fiber that is not digested. However, although these soften the stool, they are intended more for true constipation rather than that which stems from being frightened to obey the urge.

And remember – like almost everything in labor – it is never as bad again once you have managed it.

REFERENCES

AGGARWAL R, AGGARARWAL A, "Professional advice on common breast-feeding problems: a primary care study", *British Journal of General Practice*, Vol 47, No 416, March 1997, pp173–174

ALBRECHTSEN S, RASMUSSEN S et al, "Evaluation of a protocol for selecting fetuses in breech presentation for vaginal delivery or cesarean section", *American Journal of Obstetric and Gynaecology 1997*, Vol 177, No 3, Sept 1997, pp568–592

ALLOT H, PALMER C, "Sweeping the membranes: a valid procedure in stimulating the onset of labor?", *British Journal of Obstetrics and Gynaecology*, Vol 100, No 10, Oct 1993, pp893–903

ANDERSON T, "Support in Labor", *Modern Midwife*, Jan 1996, pp7–11

ANDERSON T, "Me and My Birth Ball", *Practising Midwife*, Vol 1, No 9, Sept 1998, p38

ARTSWAGER, KAY MARGARITA, *Anthropology of Human Birth*, F A Davis, 1982

ASTBURY J, "Labor pain: the role of childbirth education, information and expectation", in Peck C, Wallis M (Eds), *Problems in Pain*, Pergamon, London 1980, pp245–252

AUGUSTINSSON L, BOHLIN P, BUNDSEN P, CARLSSON C, SJOBERG P, TYREMAN N, "Pain Relief During Delivery by Transcentaneous Electrical Nerve Stimulation", *Pain*, Vol 4, 1977, pp59–65

BECK C TATANO, "Women's temporal experiences during the delivery process: a phenomenological study", *International Journal of Nursing Studies*, Vol 31, 1994, pp245–252

BECK N, HALL D, "After Office Hours: Natural Childbirth, A review and analysis", *Obstetrics and Gynaecology*, Vol 52, No 3, Sept 1978, pp371–379

BECK N, SIEGEL L, "Preparation for Childbirth and Contemporary Research on Pain, Anxiety and Stress Reduction: A Review and Critique", *Psychosomatic Medicine* Vol 42, No 4, July 1980, pp429–447

BELSEY E, ROSENBLATT D, LIEBERMAN B et al, "The influence of maternal analgesia on neonatal behavior; 1 Pethidine", *British Journal of Obstetrics and Gynaecology*, Vol 88, April 1981, pp396–406.

BIRCH E, "The experience of touch received during labor", *Journal of Nurse-Midwifery*, Vol 31, No 6, Nov–Dec 1986, pp270–276

BORELL W, FERNSTROM I, "The mechanism of labor", *Radiologic Clinics of North America*, Vol 5, No 73, 1966

BRIGHAM M, "Mothers' report of the outcome of nipple shield use", *Journal of Human Lactation*, Vol 12, No 4, Dec 1996, pp291–297

BROWN S, CAMBBELL D, KURTZ A, "Characteristics of labor pain at two stages of cervical dilation", *Pain,* Vol 38, 1989, pp289–295

BUDD S, in *Complementary Therapies in Pregnancy and Childbirth*, Tiran and Mack (Eds), 1995

BURKE E, KILFOYLE A, "A Comparative Study Waterbirth and Bedbirth", *Midwives*, Jan 1995, pp3–7

CAMMU H, CLASEN K, VAN WETTEREL et al, "To bathe or not to bathe during the first stage of labor", *Acta Obstetrica Gynaecologica Scandinavia*, Vol 73, 1994, pp468–472

CARROLL D, MOORE R, TRAMER M et al, *Contemporary Reviews in Obstetrics and Gynecology*, Vol 9, No 3, Sept 1997, pp195–205

CHIPPINGTON DERRICK D, LOWDON G, BARLOW F, *Cesarean Birth–your questions answered*, National Childbirth Trust, London, 1996

CLARK M, McCORKLER, WILLIAMS S, "Music therapy assisted labor and delivery", *Journal of Music Therapy*, Vol 18, No 2, 1981, pp88–100

COGAN R, "Effects of Childbirth Preparation", *Clinical Obstetrics and Gynecology*, Vol 23, No 1, Mar 1980, pp1–14

CONSTANTINE G, LUESLEY D, REDMAN C, O'CONNOR A, "Racial variations in the choice of analgesia in labor", *Journal of Obstetrics and Gynaecology*, Vol 9, 1989, pp189–192

COTTEN S, "Strategies for Labor Pain Relief – Past, Present and Future", *Acta Anaesthesiologica Scandinavia*, 1997, pp17–21

CRAFTER H, "Pain-free labor?", *Nursing Times*, Vol 85, No 20, 17 May 1989, pp66–68

CROWE K, VON BAEYER C, "Predictors of a Positive Childbirth Experience", *Birth 16*, 2 June 1989, pp59–63

DAVENPORT-SLACK B A, "Comparative evaluation of obstetrical hypnosis and ante–natal childbirth training", *International Journal of Clinical and Experimental Hypnosis*, Vol 23, 1975, pp266–28

DAVIES J, HEY E, REID W et al, "Prospective regional study of planned home births", *British Medical Journal*, Vol 313, No 7068, 23 Nov 1996, pp1302–1306

DEPARTMENT OF HEALTH, "NHS Maternity Statistics, England 1989–90 to 1994–5", Department of Health, London, 1997

DEWAN G, GLAZENER C, TUNSTALL M, "Postnatal pain: a neglected area" *British Journal of Midwifery*, Vol 1, No 2, June 1993, pp63–66

EGGERS P, "Pain is not a four-letter word", *International Journal of Childbirth Educators*, Vol 10, No 4, pp4–5

ENGLEMANN G, *Labor among Primitive People*, 2nd Edn. J H Chambers and Co, St Louis or New York, AMS Press, 1882

ENKIN M, KEIRSE M, RENFREW M, NEILSON J, *A Guide to Effective Care in Pregnancy and Childbirth*, 2nd Edn, Oxford University Press, Oxford, 1995

ERIKSSON M, LADFORS L, MATTSON L–A et al, "Warm tub bath during labor: A study of 1385 women with prelabor rupture of the membranes after 34 weeks of gestation", *Acta Obstetricia Scandinavia*, Vol 75, No 7, Aug 1996, pp642–644

FEN CHEUNG N, "Pain in Normal Labor. A Comparison of Experiences in Southern China and Scotland", *Midwives Chronicle and Nursing Notes*, June 1994, pp212–216

FISK K, "The Transcendent Quality of Pain in Childbirth", *Mothering*, Spring 1997, pp57–60

FLEMING A, RUBLE D, ANDERSON V. "Place of childbirth intervenes feelings of satisfaction and control in first time mothers", *Journal of Psychosomatic Obstetrics and Gynaecology*, Vol 8, No 1, Feb 1988, pp1–17

FOSTER J, SWEENEY B, "The Mechanisms of Acupuncture Analgesia", *British Journal of Hospital Medicine*, Oct 1987, pp308–312

FRIDH G, KOPARE T, GASTON-JOHANSSON F, NORVELL K T, "Factors Associated with More Intense Labor Pain", *Research in Nursing and Health*, Vol 11, 1988, pp117–124

FRIDH G, GASTON-JOHANSSON F, "Do primiparas and multiparas have realistic expectations of labor", *Acti Obstetrica et Gynaecologica Scandinavia*, Vol 69, No 2, 1990, pp103–109

GARCIA J, CORRY M, MACDONALD P, ELBOURNE D, GRANT A, "Mothers' Views of Continuous Electronic Fetal Heart Monitoring and Intermittent Auscultation in a Randomized Controlled Trial", *Birth*, Vol 12, No 2, Summer 1985, pp79–85

GASTON-JOHANSSON F, FRIDH G, TURNER NORVELL K, "Progression of Labor Pain in Primiparas and Multiparas", *Nursing Research*, Vol 37, No 2, Mar–Apr 1988, pp86–90

GEDEN E, LOWER M, BEATTIE S, BECK N, "Effects of Music and Imagery on Physiologic and Self-Report of Analogued Labor Pain", *Nursing Research*, Vol 38, No 1, Jan/Feb 1989, pp37–41

GÉLIS, JACQUES, translated by Morris, R, *A History of Childbirth – fertility, pregnancy and birth in early modern Europe*, Polity Press, 1991

GOLAY J, VEDAM S, SORGER L, "The Squatting Position for the Second Stage of Labor: Effects on Labor and on Material and Fetal Well–Being", *Birth*, Vol 20, No 2, Jun 1993, pp73–79

GRANT J M, *British Journal of Obstetrics and Gynaecology*, Vol 100, No 10, Oct 1993, pp889–90

GREEN J, "Expectations and Experiences of Pain in Labor: Findings from a Large Prospective Study" *Birth*, Vol 20, No 2, Jun 1993, pp65–72

HALLDORSDOTTIR S, KARLSDOTTIR S I, "Journeying Through Labor and Delivery: Perceptions of Women Who Have Given Birth", *Midwifery*, Vol 12, 1996, pp48–61

HANSER S, LARSON S, O'CONNELL A, "The effects of music on relaxation of expectant mothers during labor", *Journal of Music Therapy*, Vol 20, No 2, 1983, pp50–59

HAPIDOU E, DECATANZARO D, "Responsive to Laboratory Pain in Woman as a Function of Age and Childbirth Pain Experience", *Pain*, Vol 48, 1992, pp177–181

HARMON T, HYNAN M, TYRE T, "Improved obstetric outcome using hypnotic analgesia and skill mastery combined with childbirth education", *Journal of Consulting and Clinical Psychology*, Vol 58, 1990, pp79–83

HEMMINKI E, GRAUBARD E, "Cesarean Section and Subsequent Fertility: Results from the 1982 National Survey of Family Growth", American Fertility Society, 1985

HERPOLSHEIMER A, SCHRETENTHALER J, "The Use of Intrapartum Intrathecal Narcotic Analgesia in a Community–based Hospital", *Obstetrics and Gynaecology*, Vol 84, No 6, Decr 1994, pp931–936

HEWISON A, "The Language of Labor: An Examination of the Discourses of Childbirth", *Midwifery*, Vol 9, 1993, pp225–234

HOLDCROFT A, "The Physiology and Psychology of Labor Pain: A Review", *Journal of the Association of Chartered Physiotherapists in Women's Health*, No 878, Feb 1996, pp22–24

HOLDCROFT A, MORGAN M, "An Assessment of the Analgesic Effect in Labor of Pethidrine and 50 per cent Nitrous Oxide in Oxygen (Entonox)", *The Journal of Obstetrics and Gynaecology of the British Commonwealth*, Vol 81, Aug 1974, pp603–607

HUNT S, SYMONDS A, *The Social Meaning of Midwifery*, Macmillan, London, 1995

JACOBSON B, NYBERG K et al, "Opiate Addiction in Adult Offspring through Possible Imprinting After Obstetric Treatment", *British Medical Journal*, Vol 3011, 10 Nov 1990, pp1067–1070

JIMENEZ S, "Pain and Comfort: Establishing a Common Vocabulary for Exploring Issues of Pain and Comfort", *The Journal of Perinatal Education*, Vol 5, No 3, 1996, pp53–57

JOHNSON J, "Effects of accurate expectations about sensations on the sensory components and distress components of pain", *Journal of Personality and Social Psychology*, Vol 29, 1973, pp710–718

JOHNSON J, RICE V, "Sensory and Distress Components of Pain", *Nursing Research*, Vol 23, 1974, pp203–209

JOHNSON J, RICE V, FULLER S et al, "Sensory information, instruction in coping strategy, and recovery from surgery", *Research in Nursing and Health*, Vol 1, No 1, 1978, pp4–17

JOHNSON M, "Transcutaneous Electrical Nerve Stimulation in Pain Management", *British Journal of Midwifery*, Vol 5, No 7, Jul 1997, pp400

KEPPLER A B, "The use of intravenous fluids during labor", *Birth*, Vol 15, 1988 pp75–79

KIRKHAM M, PERKINS E, *Reflections on Midwifery*, Bailliere Tindall, 1997

LANGFORD JEANNE, "Pain Relief in Labor, Dispellng the Mythology in Ante-Natal Clases", *New Generation Digest*, Vol 16, No 1, Mar 1997, pp6–7

LEDERMAN R, LEDERMAN E, WORK B, McCANN D, "Relationship of Psychological Factors in Pregnancy to Progress in Labor", *Nursing Research*, Vol 28, No 2, Mar–Apr 1979, pp94–97

LEDERMAN R, LEDERMAN E, WORK B, McCANN D, "The Relationship of Maternal Anxiety, Plasma Catecholamines, and Plasma Cortisol to Progress in Labor", *American Journal of Obstetrics and Gynecology*, Vol 132, No 495, 1978, pp495–500

LE MAY, A, "The Human Connection", *Nursing Times*, Vol 82, 19 Nov 1986, pp38–30

LENSTRUP C, SCHANTZ A, BERGET A et al, "Warm bath tub during delivery", *Acta Obstetric Gynaecologica Scandinavia*, Vol 66, 1987, pp709–712

LILFORD R, "Maternal mortality and cesarean section", *British Journal of Obstetrics and Gynaecology*, Vol 97, 1990, pp883–92

LINDQVISTA, NORDEN–LINDEBERG S, "Perinatal morality and route of delivery in term breech presentations", *British Journal of Obstetrics and Gynaecology*, Vol 104, No 11, Nov 1997, pp1288–1291

LIVINGSTON J, "Music for the childbearing family", *Journal of Obstetrics, Gynaecologic and Neonatal Nursing*, Vol 8, 1979, pp363–367

LOVENSEN M, "Effects of Touch in Patients During a Crisis Situation" in *Nursing Research: Ten Studies in Patient Care*, Wilson-Barnett (Ed), Wiley, Chichester, 1983

LOWE N K, "The Pain and Discomfort of Labor and Birth", *Journal of Obstetrics, Gynaecologic and Neonatal Nursing*, Vol 25, No 1, Jan 1996, pp82–92

LOWE, N K, "Individual Variation in Childbirth Pain", *Journal of Psychosomatic Obstetrics and Gynaecology*, Vol 7, 1987, pp183–192

LUDKA L, "Fasting during labor", MIDIRS Information Pack No 7, Apr 1988

LUMEY L, RAVELLIT A, WIESSING L, KIPPE J, TREFFERS P, STEIN Z, "The Dutch Famine Birth Cohort Study: Design, Valuation of Exposure and Selected Characteristics of Subjects after 43 Years Follow–up", *Paediatric and Perinatal Epidemiology*, Vol 7, 1993, pp354–367

LYNAM L, MILLER M A, "Mothers' and Nurses' Perceptions of the Needs of Women Experiencing Preterm Labor", *Journal of Obstetrics, Gynaecology and Neonatal Nursing*, Vol 2, No 2, Mar/Apr 1992, pp126–136

MARSHALL V, "Management of premature rupture of membranes at or near term", *Journal of Nurse-Midwifery*, Vol 38, No 3, May/Jun 1993, pp140–145

McCAY S, YAGER SMITH S, "What are they talking about? Is something wrong? Information Sharing During the Second Stage of Labor," *Birth*, Vol 20, No 3, Sept 1993, pp142–147

McKAY S, ROBERTS J, "Obstetrics by Ear. Maternal and Caregiver Perceptions of the Meaning of Maternal Sounds During Second Stage Labor", *Journal of Nurse-Midwifery*, Vol 35, No 5, Sept–Oct 1990, pp266–273

MEAD M, "The Diagnosis of Foetal Distress: A Challenge to Midwives", *Journal of Advanced Nursing*, Vol 23, 1996, pp975–983

MEH L, "Scientific research on childbirth alternatives: What can it tell us about hospital practice?", in: *21st Century Obstetrics Now*, Vol 1, Stewart and Stewart D (Eds), Marble Hill MO, NAPSAC, 1977

MELZACK K, TAENZER P, FELDMAN P, KINCH R, "Labor is Still Painful After Prepared Childbirth Training", *Canadian Medical Association Journal*, 15 Aug 1981, Vol 125, pp357–363

MERCIER F, BENHAMOU D, "Hyperthermia Related to Epidural Analgesia During Labor", *International Journal of Obstetric Anaesthesia*, Vol 6, 1997, pp19–24

MIDIRS, "Breast-feeding or bottle-feeding: informed choice for professionals", "Feeding your baby – breast or bottle – informed choice for women" Informed Choice Leaflets, 1997

MIDIRS, "Breech Baby – for women", "Breech Presentation – for professionals", Informed Choice Leaflets, Jan 1997

MITTENDORF R, WILLIAMS M, BERKEY C et al, "The length of uncomplicated human gestation", *Obstetrics and Gynaecology*, Vol 75, No 6, Jun 1990, pp929–932

MOORE S, "Pain Relief in Labor: An Overview", *British Journal of Midwifery*, Vol 2, No 10, Oct 1994, pp483–486

MORGAN B, "Changes in Attitude Towards Pain Relief in Labor", *Journal of Obstetrics and Gynaecology*, Vol 10, No 3, 1990, pp236–237

MORGAN B, "Parental Attitudes to Analgesia in Labor", *Update*, 1 Mar 1986, pp401–408

MORGAN B, "Analgesia and Satisfaction in Childbirth" (The Queen Charlottes 1000 Mother Survey), *The Lancet*, Vol 2, No 8302, 9 Oct 1982, pp808–810

MORSE J, PARK C, "Home Birth and Hospital Deliveries: A Comparison of the Perceived Painfulness of Parturition", *Research in Nursing and Health*, Vol 11, 198, pp175–181

MYERS R, MYERS S, "Use of Sedative, Analgesic and Anaesthetic Drugs During Labor and Delivery: Bane or Boon?", *American Journal of Obstetrics and Gynecology*, Vol 133, No 1, 1 Jan 1979, pp83–1

NELSON M, "Working-class Women, Middle-class Women, and Models of Childbirth", *Social Problems*, Vol 30, No 3, Feb 1983

NELSSON-RYAN S, "Positioning: Second Stage Labor" in: *Childbirth Education: Practice, Research Theory*, Nichols F, Humenick S (Eds), Saunders, Philadelphia, 1989, pp256–274

NEWMARK J, HAMMERLE A, BIEGELMAYER C H, "Effects of Epidural Anaesthesia on Plasma Catecholomines and Cortisol in Parturition", *Acta Anaesthesiologica Scandinavia*, Vol 29, 4, pp555–559

NEWTON C, "Patient's knowledge of aspects of labor", *Nursing Times*, Vol 87, No 12, 20 Mar 1991, p50

NEWTON N, PEELER D , NEWTON M, "Effect of Disturbance on Labor", *American Journal of Obstetrics and Gynecology*, Vol 101, No 8, 15 Aug 1968, pp1096–1102

NEWTON N, FOSHEE D, NEWTON M, "Experimental Inhibition of Labor Through Environmental Disturbance", *Obstetrics and Gynecology*, Vol 27, No 3, Mar 1966, pp371–377

NIVEN C, "Memory for Labor Pain: Context and Quality", *Pain*, Vol 64, No 2, Feb 1995, pp387–392

NIVEN C, "Labor Pain: Long-term Recall and Consequences", *Journal of Reproductive and Infant Psychology*, Vol 6, No 2, 1988, pp83–87

ODENT M, "Can Research be Politically Incorrect?", *Midwifery Today*, Spring 1998, pp31–32

OLOFSSON C, EKBLOM A et al, "Lack of analgesic effect of systemically administered morphine or Pethidine on labor pain", *British Journal of Obstetrics and Gynaecology*, Vol 103, No 10, Oct 1996, pp968–972

ORLEANS M, "Lessons from the Dublin study of electronic fetal monitoring", *Birth*, Vol 12 , No 2, Summer 1985, pp86

PENGELLY L, GYTE G, "Briefing on Eating and Drinking in Labor" leaflet, National Childbirth Trust, 1996

PITCOCK C D H, "From Fanny to Fernand: The development of consumerism in pain control during the birth process", *American Journal of Obstetrics and Gynecology*, Vol 167, No 3, Sept 1992, pp581–587

PRICE S, "Birth plans and their impact on midwifery care", *MDIRS Midwifery Digest*, Vol 8, No 2, Jun 1998, pp189–191

RAJAN L, "Perceptions of pain and pain relief in labor: the gulf between experience and observation", *Midwifery*, Vol 3, 1993, pp136–45,

RAJAN LYNDA, "The impact of obstetric procedures and analgesia/anaesthesia during labor and delivery on breast feeding", *Midwifery*, Vol 10, 1994, pp87–103

REYNOLDS F, CROWHURST J, "Opioids in Labor – no analgesic effort", *The Lancet*, Vol 349, 4 Jan 1997, p4–5

ROBERTSON A, *Empowering Women: Teaching Active Birth in the '90s*, Ace Graphics, Sydney, 1994

ROBERTSON A, *Preparing for Birth: Background Notes for Pre-Natal Classes*, ACE Graphics, Sydney, 1993

ROSENBLATT D, BELSEY E, LIEBEMAN B, REDSHAW M, et al, "The Influence of Maternal Analgesia on Neonatal Behaviours II Epidural Bupivicaine," *British Journal of Obstetrics and Gynaecology*, Vol 88, Apr 1981, pp407–413

RUBIN R, "Maternal Touch", *Nursing Outlook*, Vol 11, 1963, pp828–831

SAMMONS L, "The use of music by women during childbirth", *Journal of Nurse-Midwifery*, Vol 29, 1985, pp266–270

SANDER H, GINTZLER A, "Spinal cord mediation of the opioid analgesia of pregnancy", *Brain Research*, Vol 408, 1987, pp389–393

SAUNDERS N, PATERSON C, "Can we abandon Naegele's rule?", *The Lancet*, Vol 337, 9 Mar 1991

SCHIFF E, FRIEDMAN S, "Maternal and neonatal outcome of 846 term singleton breech deliveries seven year experience at a single center", *American Journal of Obstetrics and Gynecology*, Vol 175, No 1, Jul 1996, pp18–23

SCHROEDER C, ROBERTS J, "The Technical versus the Relational Approach to Women's Pain in Childbirth", In: Proceedings of the International Confederation of Midwives, 23rd International Congress 1993, Vancouver ICM, Vol IV, 1993, pp1652–1671

SHANLEY L K, "Love is the heart of labor", *Midwifery Today*, No 31, Autumn 1994, pp17–18

SHAPIRO M, NAJMAN A, CHANG A et al, "Information control and the exercise of power in the obstetrical encounter", *Social Science and Medicine*, Vol 17, N. 3, 1083, pp139–146

SHARMA J, NEWMAN M et al, "National Audit on the practice and training in breech deliveries in the United Kingdom", *International Journal of Gynaecology and Obstetrics*, Vol 59, No 2, Nov 1997, pp103–108

SHIPMAN M, BONIFACE D, TEFFT M, "Antenatal perineal massage and subsequent perineal outcomes: a randomised controlled trial" *British Journal of Obstetrics and Gynaecology*, Vol 104, No 7, Jul 1997, pp787–791

SIMKIN P, "Just Another Day in a Woman's Life? Women's Long-Term Perceptions of Their First Birth Experience, Part I", *Birth*, Vol 18, No 4, Dec 1991, pp203–210

SIMKIN P, "Just Another Day in a Woman's Life? Part II: Nature and Consistency of Women's Long-Term Memories of the First Birth Experiences", *Birth*, Vol 19, No 2, Jun 1992, pp64–81

SIMKIN P, "Stress, Pain and Catecholomines in Labor: Part 1, A Review", *Birth*, Vol 13, No 4, Dec 1986, pp227–233

SJOGREN B, *MIDIRS Midwifery Digest*, June 1998, page 172

SKIBSTED L, LANGE A, "The need for pain relief in uncomplicated deliveries in an alternative birth center compared to an obstetric delivery ward", *Pain*, Vol 48, 1992, pp183–186

SLADE P, MACPHERSON P, HUME A, MARESH M, "Expectations, experiences and satisfaction with labor", *Journal of Clinical Psychology*, Vol 32, 1993, pp469–483

SOSA R, KENNELL J, KLAUS M, ROBERTSON S, URRUTIA J, "The effect of a supportive companion on perinatal problems, length of labor, and mother-infant interaction", *The New England Journal of Medicine*, Vol 303, No 11, 11 Sept 1980, pp597–600

STANDLEY J, "Music research in medical/dental treatment, meta-analysis and clinical applications", *Journal of Music Therapy*, Vol 23, No 2, 1986, pp56–122

STEWART D, "Psychiatric symptoms following attempted natural childbirth", *Canadian Medical Association Journal*, Vol 127, 15 Oct 1982, pp713–716

STOLLE K, "A comparison of women's expectations of labor with the actual event", *Birth*, Vol 14, No 2, June 1987, pp93–103

TEW M, "There's no place like home", *Midwives Chronicle*, Dec 1987, p398

TEW M, "From budget to babies", *British Medical Journal*, 7 May 1988, p1333

TEW M, "Place of birth and perinatal mortality," *Journal of The Royal College of General Practitioners*, August 1985, pp390–3

TEW M, "We have the technology", *Nursing Times*, 20 Nov 1985, pp22–24

TEW M, "Do obstetric intranatal interventions make birth safer?", *British Journal of Obstetrics and Gynaecology*, July 1986, pp659–74

TEW M, "Home, hospital or bathroom?", *The Lancet*, 27 Sept 1986, pp749

TEW M, "The safest place of birth: further evidence", *The Lancet*, 30 June 1979, pp1388–90

TEW M, "Perinatal mortality: Is home a safe place?", *Health & Social Service Journal*, 30 May 1980, pp702–5

TEW M, "Where to be born", *New Society*, 20 Jan 1977, pp120–121

TEW M, "Home versus hospital confinements: the statistics", *Update*, Vol 18, 1979, pp1317–22

THACKER S B, STROUP D F, "Continuous Electronic Fetal Heart Monitoring during Labor (Cochrane Review)" in: The Cochrane Library Issue 2, Oxford: Update Software, 1998

THOMSON A, HILLIER V, "A re-evaluation of the effect of Pethidine on the length of labor", *Journal of Advanced Nursing*, Vol 19, 1994, pp448–456

THORNTON J, LILFORD R, "Active management of labor – current knowledge and research issues", *British Medical Journal*, Vol 309, 6 Aug 1994, pp366–369

VARRASS G, BAZZANO C, EDWARDS W T, "Effects of physical activity on maternal plasma beta-endorphin levels and perception of labor pain", *American Journal of Obstetrics and Gynecology*, Vol 160, No 3, Mar 1989, pp707–712

WEBER S, "Cultural aspects of pain in childbearing women", *Journal of Gynaecology, Obstetrics and Neonatal Nursing*, Vol 25, No 1, Jan 1996, pp67–72

WEINER P, HOGG M, ROSEN M, "Effects of Naloxone on Pethidine-induced neonatal depression. Part 1, Intravenous Naloxone", *British Medical Journal*, 1977, Vol 2, pp228–231

WHIPPLE B, JOSIMOVICH J, KOMISARUK B, "Sensory thresholds during the antepartum, intrapartum and postpartum periods", *International Journal of Nursing Studies*, Vol 27, No 3, 1990, pp213–221

WILSON-CLAY B, BRIGHAM M, "Clinical use of silicone nipple shields", *Journal of Human Lactation*, Vol 12, No 4, Dec 1996, pp279–285

WORLD HEALTH ORGANISATION, "Appropriate technology for birth", Lancet ii, 1985, pp436–7

WUITCHIK M, BAKALD A, LIPSHITZ J, "The clinical significance of pain and cogniture activity in latent labor", *Obstetrics and Gynaecology*, Vol 73, pp35–41

YOUNG J, "Relaxation of the pelvic joints in pregnancy: Pelvic arthropathy of pregnancy", *Journal of Obstetrics and Gynaecology of the British Empire*, Vol 47, 1940, p493

Suggested Reading

Arms, Suzanne. *Immaculate Deception II: Myth, Magic, and Birth.* Berkeley: Celestial Arts, 1994.

Balaskas, Janet and Gayle Petersen. *New Natural Pregnancy: Practical Wellbeing from Conception to Birth.* Northampton, Ma.: Interlink, 1999.

Boston Women's Health Book Collective. *Our Bodies, Ourselves for the New Century.* New York: Touchstone, 1998.

Davis, Elizabeth. *Heart & Hands: A Midwife's Guide to Pregnancy & Birth.* Rev. ed. Berkeley: Celestial Arts, 1997.

England, Allison. *Aromatherapy and Massage for Mother and Baby.* Rochester, Vt.: Healing Arts Press, 2000.

Gladstar, Rosemary. *Herbal Healing for Women: Simple Home Remedies for Women of All Ages.* New York: Simon & Schuster, 1993.

Hansen, Maren Tonder. *Mother Mysteries.* Boston: Shambhala, 1997.

Kitzinger, Sheila. *The Complete Book of Pregnancy and Childbirth.* Rev. ed. New York: Knopf, 1996.

Klaus, Marshall H.; Phyllis H. Klaus; and John Kennell. *Mothering the Mother: How a Doula Can Help You Have a Shorter, Easier, and Healthier Birth.* New York: Perseus, 1993.

Northrup, Christiane. *Women's Bodies, Women's Wisdom: Creating Physical and Emotional Health and Healing.* Rev. ed. New York: Bantam Doubleday Dell, 1998.

Stillerman, Elaine and Diana Kurz. *Mother Massage: A Handbook for Relieving the Discomforts of Pregnancy.* New York: Delta, 1994.

Tyler, Varro E. *The Honest Herbal: A Sensible Guide to the Use of Herbs and Related Remedies.* New York: Pharmaceutical Products Press, 1993.

Weed, Susun S. *The Wisewoman Herbal for the Childbearing Year.* Woodstock, N.Y.: Ash Tree Publishing, 1986.

Wesson, Nicky. *Home Birth.* London: Vermilion, 1996.

———. *Natural Mothering.* Rochester, Vt.: Healing Arts Press, 1997.

Wildwood, Chrissie. *The Encyclopedia of Aromatherapy.* Rochester, Vt.: Healing Arts Press, 1997.

Ullman, Dana. *The Consumers' Guide to Homeopathy.* New York: Putnam, 1995.

RESOURCES

General
Doulas of North America (DONA)
13513 North Grove Drive
Alpine, UT 84004
(801) 756-7331
www.dona.com

Global Maternal/Child Health
Association
Waterbirth International
P.O. Box 1400
Wilsonville, OR 97070
(503) 682-3600
www.geocities.com/Hot Springs/2840

Midwives Alliance of North America
(MANA)
P.O. Box 175
Newton, KS 67114
(888) 923-6262
www.mana.org

Childbirth and Postpartum
Professionals Association (CAPPA)
310 Sweet Ivy Lane
Lawrenceville, GA 30043
(888) 548-3672
www.postpartumdoula.com

Cesarean/Support, Education, and
Concern (C/SEC)
22 Forest Road
Framingham, MA 01701
(508) 877-8266

Acupuncture
American Academy of Medical
Acupuncture (AAMA)
Administrative Offices
5820 Wilshire Boulevard, Suite 500
Los Angeles, CA 90036
(323) 937-5514
www.medicalacupuncture.org

Aromatherapy
Aroma Vera, Inc.
5901 Rodeo Road
Los Angeles, CA 90016-4312
(800) 669-9514

Herbal Medicine
Herb Research Foundation
1007 Pearl Street, Suite 200
Boulder, CO 80302
(303) 449-2265
www.herbs.org

Homeopathy
Nelson Bach USA
Wilmington Technology Park
100 Research Drive
Wilmington, MA 01887-4406
(800) 319-9151
www.nelsonbach.com

Hypnotherapy
American Council of Hypnotist
Examiners
700 South Central Avenue
Glendale, CA 91204-2011
(818) 242-1159
www.sonic.net/hypno/ache.html

INDEX

acetaminophen, 5, 9, 139–40
acupressure (shiatsu), 103, 109–11
acupuncture, 38, 66, 103, 105–7
adrenaline, 3, 31, 114
afterpains, 105, 139
alternative birth center (ABC), 46
ambulance, calling, 10, 11
amniotic fluid, 4, 6–7, 16, 34, 87
amniotomy, 35
anesthetic, general, 17, 73, 133
antibiotics, 8, 24
anxiety, 20, 22–23, 26–27, 31–32, 41, 56
Apgar scores, 119
ARM. see membranes, artificial rupture
Arnica, 99, 103, 129, 139
aromatherapy, 94–98

baby
    altering position, 65–66, 81, 105
    decrease in movement, 4, 33
    drug effects, 18, 35, 119, 124–25
    head emergence, 16, 63
    head not engaged, 7, 65
    oxygen supply, 7, 78, 79, 82, 83, 114, 131
    positions, 7, 30, 61–66, 131
    stress hormones, 32–33
backache, 1, 6, 64, 65, 124, 137
backache remedies, 95, 103, 105, 112
bag, packing, 57, 75–77
bathing, 8, 13, 43, 56, 65, 86
belt monitor, 81, 82–83
birth
    predicted date, 1–2, 34,36
    satisfaction with, 18, 124
birth ball, 13, 68, 81

birth partners, 57–61
    home births, 51
    hospital births, 12, 42, 57–59
    how to help, 41, 59–60, 70–71, 80
    making decisions, 21, 60–61, 66
birth plans, 12, 57, 66–68, 75, 127
birth supporters, 19, 41–42, 54–57
birthing chairs, 79–80
bladder
    emptying, 12, 56, 59
    pressure on, 30, 65
bleeding
    birthing chairs, 80
    early labor, 5, 10
    postpartum, 138–39
    third stage of labor, 17
    transition/second stage, 14
blood pressure
    high, 24, 31, 33, 131
    low, 15, 78, 79, 123
bowels, emptying of, 4, 139–40
Braxton-Hicks contractions, 5–6, 29, 70
breast milk
    acupuncture, 107
    laxative excretion, 140
    let-down reflex, 3
breastfeeding
    birth supporters, 56, 128
    cesarean section, 133
    Demerol in baby, 119
    episiotomies, 127, 128
breathing techniques
    during labor, 13, 15, 42
    first bowel movement, 140
    reflexology, 104
    relaxation technique, 13
breech position, 7, 105
bucket, 11, 13, 77

Bupivicaine for epidurals, 122, 124–25

Cardiotocograph (CTG), 81
castor oil, 37
catecholamines, 31–33
cervix
    dilation, 5, 8, 10, 13, 14, 19, 29
    induction of labor, 34–35
    ripeness, 8, 34, 35, 37
    self-exam, 8–9
    start of contractions, 3, 4–5, 8
    sweeping/stripping, 5, 34, 37
cesarean sections, 131–35
    eating during labor, 73–74
    emergency, 73, 83, 133
    epidurals, 73, 123
    essential, 131–32
    increased numbers of, 7, 82, 131
    operation, 132–33
    post-operative care, 134–35
    prolonged induced labor, 7, 35, 36
    reasons, 62, 82, 83, 131–32
colostrum, 3
compresses, 56, 77, 96, 97, 129
constipation, 12, 95, 103, 106, 139
contractions, 3
    Braxton Hicks, 5–6, 29, 70
    early labor, 5, 8, 10–11, 43
    first stage of labor, 13, 112
    frequency, 5–6, 10
    homeopathy, 101–2
    induced labor, 35
    intensity, 5–6, 13, 19
    labor position effect, 79
    start of labor, 3, 5–6
    stress hormones, 30
    transition stage, 14
control
    drug use, 18, 60–61, 114, 119
    hypnotherapy, 115
    importance of, 39, 61
    transition stage, 14
coping strategies, 13–14, 43–44
Corcoran, Debra, 102–3
cord, 7, 11, 17, 131
Coveney, Marie, 48–50

crowning, 16, 129
cultural differences, 44–45, 54, 78, 92

Demerol, 46, 113, 118–20
diarrhea, 4, 37, 139
digestive system, 9, 31, 72, 93, 118
distraction techniques, 43–44
disturbances, 39–41
Doberska, Cathy, 38
drugs
    acceptance, 18, 60–61
    birth plan, 12
    Bupivacaine for epidurals, 122,
        124–25
    Demerol, 46, 113, 118–20
    morphine barbiturates, 119
    Narcan, as antidote, 119
due date, 1–2, 34, 36

early labor, 1–7, 9–12, 43, 65, 112
eating/drinking, 9, 12, 43, 48, 57, 59,
    72–75
EMF. see fetal Monitoring
endorphins, 30, 31, 112, 113, 136
enema, 12, 37, 140
environment, 46–53
    choosing, 20–22, 50–51
    effect on labor, 3, 11, 28, 31, 40
ephedrine, 123
epidural, 30, 122–25
    cesarean section, 132–33
    control issue, 18, 60–61
    induced labor, 36–37
    position during labor, 79
    second stage of labor, 15, 123
    TENS machine, 113
epinephrine, 31
episiotomies, 23, 127–30
Ergotrate, 17
essential oils, 93, 94, 95–96, 129
expectations, 20–22, 26–27

father of baby, 20, 45, 48, 54–55, 56
fear, 20, 23, 27, 31, 115
feet, 71, 103, 105
Ferguson's reflex, 15

fetal distress, 6–7, 32, 86, 127, 133
fetal monitoring, 12, 36
    Doppler machine, 81, 83
    electronic (EFM), 41, 48, 81–84
first stage of labor, 9, 12–14, 29, 112
forceps delivery
    birth supporter, 55
    birthing chair, 80
    epidurals, 123
    episiotomy, 127
    fetal monitoring, 82
    induced labor, 35, 37
    starvation during labor, 74

glucose drip, 74

hands, reflexology, 103, 104–5
Hargreaves, Sue, 115–17
headache, 103, 105, 106, 124
hemorrhoids, 95, 103, 106, 107
herbal medicines, 91–94, 129–30
Heywood, Karen, 24–26
home birth
    benefits, 19, 45, 48
    choosing, 3, 10, 22, 48–53
    packing bag for, 76
    pain intensity, 46–47
    risk statistics, 47
    water birth, 87
homeopathy, 98–102
    during labor, 100–102
    inducing labor, 38
    perineal damage, 129, 130
    position of baby, 66, 101
    preparing for labor, 77
hormones, 3, 4, 17, 31, 136
hospital
    admission, 41, 67
    choosing, 20–22, 57
    eating and drinking, 73
    environmental stress, 11–12, 40, 48
    infant mortality rate, 47
    length of stay, 137
    medical interventions, 23, 31, 35,
        56, 82
    trust in staff, 40
    when to go, 6, 9, 10–12, 59
hypnotherapy, 27, 115

induction, 33–38
    after membrane rupture, 7
    agreeing to, 34, 36–37
    medical procedures, 34–35
    other methods, 37–38, 105
    power of mind, 3–4
infection
    after birth, 80, 138, 139
    after membrane rupture, 7–8, 35
    in hospitals, 48
    starvation during labor, 74
irritability, 4, 14, 55, 59–60, 101

James, Jeanette, 84–85
Jones, Joan, 120–21

Kahn, Amarit, 121–22
Ketonuria, 74
knee-chest position, 65, 80
kneeling position, 68, 78

labor, 1–17
    duration, 7
    early, 1–7, 9–12, 43, 65, 112
    expectations, 20–22, 26–27, 56
    making noise during, 14, 15, 44–45
    physical support, 56, 80–81
    positions, 15–16, 78–85
    slow, 31–32, 37, 86, 104, 109–11,
        119
labor, stages of
    first, 9, 12–14, 29, 112
    second, 3, 9, 14–16, 45, 79, 114, 123
    third, 16–17
    time limits on, 14, 48
    transition, 14, 70
lochia, 136, 138–39
Long, Karen, 51–53

massage
    during labor, 13, 60, 70–72, 93,
        96–98
    inducing labor, 37

perineal, 127–29, 130
massage techniques, 71–72
meconium, 6–7, 34
membranes
    artificial rupture, 3, 7, 35, 83
    rupture, 3, 6–8, 10, 14
    sweeping/stripping, 5, 34, 37
Mendelson's syndrome, 73
midwife
    birth plans, 12, 17, 66–68
    changing, 12, 41–42, 58
    early labor, 3–4, 6, 10, 11–12
    home births, 10, 11, 48–51
    independent, 10, 41
    induced labor, 34, 37
    skills, 51, 80–81, 104, 105, 127–28
    trust in, 36, 40, 54, 58
    water births, 87
Midwives Alliance of North America,
    50
mind, influence of, 3–4, 28
mobility, 13, 42, 67, 123
Montgomery's Rule, 2

Naegele's Rule, 2
natural aids, 86–117
    acupressure, 103, 109–11
    acupuncture, 38, 103, 105–7
    aromatherapy, 94–98
    herbal medicines, 91–94, 129–30
    homeopathy, 98–102
    music, 91
    reflexology, 103–5
    water, 8, 43, 86–88
    see also TENS machine
nausea, 95, 106, 118
nipples, 37, 137
noise during labor, 14, 15, 40, 44–45
noradrenaline/norepinephine, 31, 32

obstetric interventions, 23, 31, 35, 56,
    82
occipito-anterior (OA) positions, 62–64
occipito-posterior (OP) positions, 62,
    64–66

oils, massage, 77, 93, 96, 128
oxytocin, 3
    conception, 3
    epidurals, 123
    induction of labor, 35
    occipito-posterior (OP) labor, 64
    placenta delivery, 16, 17
    pushing phase, 15
    starvation during labor, 74
    stress effect, 31, 32

pain, 18–27
    causes, 20, 29–30
    experience of pain, 9–10, 13, 30–31
    intensity, 11, 18–20, 28, 30–31
    labor position effect, 79
    minimization of, 24, 42–45
    postpartum, 105, 127–28, 136–40
    psychological, 20
    see also drugs; natural aids
pelvis, rocking, 65
Pentesco-Gilbert, Deborah, 88–90
perineum
    damage, 56, 80, 127–30, 139–40
    message, 127–29, 130
    pain during labor, 9, 16, 29, 112
    pushing phase, 15, 16
placenta
    blocking cervix, 131
    expulsion, 16–17
    premature detachment, 5, 10, 131
    retained, 105, 107, 111
position
    of baby, 7, 30, 35, 61–66, 127
    changing, 15–16, 42, 56, 59
postmaturity, 33–34
postnatal depression, 56, 105, 107
postpartum hemorrhage, 111, 138
postpartum pain, 105, 127–28, 136–40
preeclampsia, 33, 131
pregnancy
    endorphin levels, 30
    options and expectations, 20–22
    substances to avoid, 94, 98
    term, 2, 4–5, 74

premature labor, 6, 111, 127, 132
prenatal classes, 23–24, 27, 68
prostaglandin, 3, 30, 34, 37
pushing phase, 14–16, 45, 79

recumbent position, 78–79, 83
reflexology, 103–5
relaxation, 13, 24, 68–70, 114–15
Rescue Remedy, Bach flower, 102
Rh (Rhesus) incompatibility, 33

second stage of labor, 3
    epidurals, 15, 123
    pain, 9, 79, 114
    pushing phase, 14–16, 45, 79
self-hypnosis, 114–15
semi-recumbent position, 78–79
sexual intercourse, 5, 8, 37, 130
show, 4–5
sitting position, 78
sleep problems, 9, 103, 104, 136–37
squatting position, 78, 80
start of labor, 3, 4, 5–6, 8, 111
starvation, during labor, 73–74
stress hormones, 31–33
Syntocinon, 17

tearing, 80, 127–30
teas, herbal, 77, 92–93
TENS machine, 111–14
    acupuncture points, 105–6, 112
    attaching, 77, 112–13
    cesarean section, 134
    early labor, 6, 11, 29, 111, 112

occipito-posterior (OP) labor, 64
    with other pain relief, 113–14
third stage of labor, 16–17
thrombosis, 137
touch, 13, 70
toxemia. see preeclampsia
Transcutaneous Electronic Nerve
    Stimulator. see TENS machine
transition stage, 14, 70
transverse position, 7, 131

ultrasound, 2, 129, 132
upright position, 15, 42, 68, 78–81
uterus
    afterpains, 105, 139
    blood flow, 15, 31, 32
    labor position effect, 79
    transition stage, 14

vaginal examinations, 8–9, 34, 37, 41
vaporization, 96
vernix, 16
visualisation, 43–44, 65, 91
vomiting, 73, 95, 106, 118

walking, 42, 43, 60
water, use during labor, 8, 43, 86–88
water birth, 8, 87
waters, breaking. see membranes
weight loss, 4
Weston, Sue, 125–26
World Health Organization, 92, 131

yoga, 24, 66